中华传统经典养生术

（汉英对照）

(Chinese- English) Traditional and Classical Chinese Health Cultivation

Chief Producer Li Jie	总策划　李　洁
Chief Compilers Li Jie Xu Feng Xiao Bin Zhao Xiaoting	总主编　李　洁　许　峰　肖　斌　赵晓霆
Chief Translator Han Chouping	总主译　韩丑萍
English Language Reviewer Lawrence Lau	英译主审　劳伦斯·刘

松柔功

Song Rou Gong (Soft and Relaxed Exercise)

编著　肖　斌
Compiler　Xiao Bin

翻译　韩丑萍
Translator　Han Chouping

上海科学技术出版社
Shanghai Scientific & Technical Publishers

图书在版编目（CIP）数据

松柔功：汉英对照 / 肖斌编著；韩丑萍译.—上
海：上海科学技术出版社，2015.5
（中华传统经典养生术）
ISBN 978-7-5478-2561-7

Ⅰ.①松… Ⅱ.①肖… ②韩… Ⅲ.①气功–健身运
动–基本知识–汉、英 Ⅳ.①R214

中国版本图书馆CIP数据核字（2015）第042964号

松柔功

编者 肖 斌

上海世纪出版股份有限公司
上 海 科 学 技 术 出 版 社 出版
中国图书进出口上海公司 发行

2015年5月第1版
ISBN 978-7-5478-2561-7/R·879

Song Rou Gong (Soft and Relaxed Exercise) · 松 柔 功

顾问委员会
Advisory Committee Members

主任

徐建光　陈凯先　严世芸　郑　锦

Directors

Xu Jianguang Chen Kaixian Yan Shiyun Zheng Jin

副主任

施建蓉　胡鸿毅　季　光　张怀琼　余小明　劳力行

Vice Directors

Shi Jianrong　Hu Hongyi　Ji Guang　Zhang Huaiqiong

Yu Xiaoming　Lao Lixing

学术顾问

严世芸　林中鹏　林　欣　李　鼎　俞尔科　王庆其
潘华信　潘华敏　姚玮莉　赵致平　李　磊

Academic Advisers

Yan Shiyun　　Lin Zhongpeng　　Shin Lin　　　Li Ding　　Yu Erke

Wang Qingqi　Pan Huaxin　　　Pan Huamin　Yao Weili

Zhao Zhiping　Li Lei

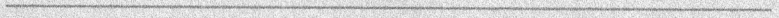

编纂委员会
Compilation Committee Members

总策划

李 洁

Chief Producer

Li Jie

总主编

李 洁 许 峰 肖 斌 赵晓霆

Chief Compilers

Li Jie Xu Feng Xiao Bin Zhao Xiaoting

副总主编

孙 磊 陈昌乐 倪青根

Vice Chief Compilers

Sun Lei Chen Changle Ni Qinggen

总主译

韩丑萍

Chief Translator

Han Chouping

副主译

赵海磊

Vice Chief Translator

Zhao Hailei

项目资助

Acknowledgement

· 上海市新闻出版专项扶持资金项目

· 上海市中医药三年行动计划（2015—2018年）"基于〈中华气功史陈列馆〉科普教育基地为核心的〈中医气功文化平台〉建设"
（项目编号: ZY3–WHJS–1–1010）

· Shanghai Press and Publication of special support funds program

· The Three-Year Action Plan for Chinese Medicine in Shanghai (2015–2018) on Construction of Qigong Cultural Platform in the Museum of Chinese Qigong History (Program No: ZY3–WHJS–1–1010)

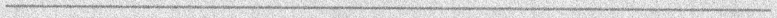

序
Foreword

欣闻上海市气功研究所编写的《中华传统经典养生术》丛书即将出版，这是中华原创医学文明传播的一件盛事，特致贺忱。

中华传统养生术源远流长，其中导引术更是重要的组成部分，它先于针、灸、药、医而形成，是中华民族最早用以防治疾病、养生保健的重要方法之一。现存早期文献《庄子》《吕氏春秋》《黄帝内经》以及考古发现《引书》《导引图》中均有关于养生导引及其具体方法的记载。此后绵绵数千年的历史长河中，中华养生导引术不断丰富、发展与创新，在自我实践中形成千门万法，在去伪存真中完善理论体系。20世纪后叶，古之导引术又以现代"气功"的面目再次席卷中华大地，并享誉海内外。时至今天，中华导引术仍然以其"人天合一"的整体观思想与丰富多姿的养生导引方法独立于世界自然医药之林，滋润着人类身心世界。事实表明，中华导引术已经形成为一门博大精深的学术体系。它所研究的是人之物质基础（精）与自组织能力（神）相互关系的规律，是关于"人"——这个地球上最复杂系统达到和谐与协调的一门学问。

我和上海市气功研究所相识逾30年，该所自20世纪70年代的中医研究所开始，气功与导引就是关注、研究的重点领域；80年代中期更名气功研究所后，更是全力着眼于现代气功的研究与中华导引术的弘扬。《中华传统经典养生术》是上海市气功研究所多年来所教授养生导引术、气功功法的汇编与总结，对于帮助学习、普及推广现代导引术具有较好的价值。希望此丛书的出版，能够进一步带动当前养生导引术在海内外的健康发展，推动中华优秀文化走向世界各地。

是以为序。

林中鹏

2015年3月

It is with great pleasure that I learn the *Traditional and Classical Chinese Health Cultivation* series compiled by the Shanghai Qigong Research Institute will be published soon. This means a lot to the spread of Chinese medical civilization.

Traditional Chinese health cultivation has a long-standing and well-established history. As an important part of health cultivation practice, Dao Yin exercise was used for disease prevention and treatment as well as life cultivation before acupuncture, moxibustion and herbal medicine. The recordings of *Dao Yin* and its specific exercise methods can be traced back to the *Zhuangzi, Lü Shi Chun Qiu* (The Annals of Lü Buwei), *Huang Di Nei Jing* (the Yellow Emperor's Inner Classic) and archaeologically unearthed books such as *Yin Shu* (a book on Dao Yin) and *Dao Yin Tu* (Dao Yin Diagram). After this, the thousands of years have witnessed the enrichment, progress and innovation of Chinese *Dao Yin* practice, coupled with emergence of numerous methods and perfection of its theoretical system. In late 20th century, the ancient *Dao Yin* exercise became exceptionally popular across China in the form of 'qigong'. Today, Chinese *Dao Yin* exercise remains flourish with its holistic 'Man-Nature Unity' idea and various exercise methods that benefit both body and mind. Facts show that there is a profound academic system behind Chinese *Dao Yin* exercise. This system studies the interactions between material foundation (essence) and self-organization ability (mind). In other words, it studies the way to achieve harmony and coordination of human being—the most complex system on earth.

I've established a friendship with the Shanghai Qigong Research Institute for 30 years. Ever since its founding in 1970s as a Research Institute of Chinese Medicine, qigong and *Dao Yin* have always been the research priorities of the Institute. The focuses on qigong and *Dao Yin* have been more highlighted in 1980s when the Institute was renamed as a Qigong Research Institute. I firmly believe that the

Traditional and Classical Chinese Health Cultivation series are of great significance in popularizing modern *Dao Yin* exercise. I sincerely wish the book series can further promote *Dao Yin* exercise at home and abroad and spread excellent Chinese culture.

For this, I wrote this forward.

Lin Zhongpeng
March 2015

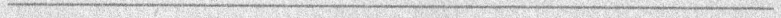

前 言
Preface

气 以 臻 道

农历乙未早春，正是上海市气功研究所创建三十周年之际，恰逢气功学术发展枯木迎春之季。在此，我们谨向海内外气功学界发出倡言——构建现代气功"气以臻道"的学术思想。

所谓"气以臻道"，首先是指气功学术发展必须树立一个大方向，即中华传统文化精神的最高目标——"道"；其次是指通过对"气"的感性体验与理性认知，使生命更趋向"道"，与"道"合一。道者，规律、目标也；气者，方法、途径也；臻者，趋向、完善也。气-道共同构成"气以臻道"学术思想内核。其中气为实、主行，是具体之指；道为虚、主理，是抽象之喻。气因道而展，道由气而实；气以道归，道以气显；气借道而实际指归，道假气而理性论证。气功学术发展必须气、道并重，互印互证，理行一贯。两者既各尽其责、各擅其能，又有主从之别。"道"因标指形上本体而为万法归宗之源；"气"每描述形下万法而成法法生灭之流。"道"经思维抽象提炼，揭示规律、规则之理性思辨；"气"常直叙主观感觉，表述体会、觉受的感性认识。道-气，一主一从，一虚一实，构成中华气功学术思想的本质内涵。

"气以臻道"学术思想之主体是"道"，是指向真理之道路，是学术文化人文精神的体现，也是先人用身心去实践生命运化规律的心得体验，古人称为"内证之学"。"道"的外延旁及"功"和"术"，可以包括各种神秘现象、气功现象、特异现象，古人称为"神通法术"。当今，现代科学研究介入传统气功学术是时代进步的表现，它为我们观察生命奥秘打开了一个全新的视角。透过唯象的研究，重新激发起人类对生命的思考与敬重，重新挖掘出科技文明下的人文精神，而非单纯地将生命物质化，这才是现代科学介入传统气功的人文价值所在。

　　有鉴于此，我们倡议构建现代气功研究之"气以臻道"学术思想，让中华传统文化与现代科学携起手来，揭示生命真谛，回归大道本源。

上海市气功研究所

2015年春

Advocacy for *Qi-Dao Harmony* in Modern Qigong Practice

　　The year 2015 is a Chinese new year of yin wood sheep (*Yi Wei* in Chinese). Wood, in Chinese culture on five elements (*Wu Xing*), is connected to the season of spring. The year 2015 also marks the 30th anniversary of the founding of Shanghai Qigong Research Institute. With a strong belief that the spring of 2015 will bring new hope to qigong study, we hereby advocate the concept of 'Qi-*Dao Harmony*' for its academic advance.

　　The term *Qi-Dao Harmony* has two underlying implications. First, it implies that *dao* is the ultimate goal of traditional Chinese culture and the general orientation for academic qigong advance. Second, it implies that our lives shall combine into one with the *dao* through perception and understanding of qi. In summary, this term means to achieve and perfect *dao* through qi exercise. The 'qi' here is weighted and refers to practice. The '*dao*' here is unweighted and refers to principles. Without *dao*, qi cannot extend; without qi, *dao* cannot become weighted. Qi finds its origin in *dao* and *dao* manifests itself in qi. Qi returns to *dao* eventually and *dao* supports qi theoretically. It's essential for people in academic qigong field to pay equal attention to qi and *dao*. The two have a principal-subordinate relationship. The metaphysical *dao* is the origin of all methods. The physical qi is the practice of all methods. *Dao* is about the abstract thinking and reveals the laws and rules. Qi is about the subjective feelings and tells experience and perception. Qi and *dao* constitute the essence of academic idea in Chinese qigong.

Let's get a deeper look into the concept of *Qi-Dao Harmony*. Also known as the 'learning of internal evidence', *dao* is the way to truth. It contains humanistic spirit and physical and mental experience of our ancestors. *Dao* extends to exercise (*gong*) and a variety of magic arts including mysterious, qigong and extrasensory phenomena. Today, modern scientific qigong research offers a new insight into the mysteries of life. The phenomenological research rekindles our reflection and respect towards life and enables us to re-discover humanism from modern civilization greatly impacted by science and technology. This is the real value of scientific research on traditional qigong in this materialized world.

To this end, we advocate the academic concept of '*Qi-Dao Harmony*' in modern qigong research. We believe the combination of traditional Chinese culture and modern science can help us to reveal the truth of life and return to the origin of the great *dao*.

Shanghai Qigong Research Institute
Spring 2015

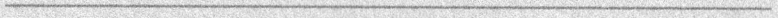

编写说明

Words from the Compilers

中华传统养生术根植于中国传统哲学、中医学和养生学,是人体自我身心锻炼的有效方法。

随着倡导"主动健康"概念日益深入人心,具有调身、调息、调心功能的中华传统养生术,以其传统的养修理论、独特的身心效果蜚声海内外,引起世人的广泛关注。但近期国内外少见中国传统养生术的书籍出版,尤其没有成套、成系列的经典养生类作品问世,更缺乏英汉对照的专业著作。

上海中医药大学上海市气功研究所研究人员在前期研究工作基础上,精选中华传统经典养生术共八种,从历史源流、功法理论、特色要领、图解动作、分解说明与具体运用几方面进行中文编纂,由上海中医药大学中医英语专业人员进行翻译。并邀请专家进行中文审稿,邀请美国友三中医药大学Lawrence Lau先生审定英文翻译。

本套丛书详细地将八种中华经典养生术以图文并茂、视频摄像的形式记录下来,配以光盘,非常方便学习与传播,尤其便于海外养生爱好者以英语来学习。

本套丛书编纂过程中,得到上海市中医药三年行动计划(2015—2018年)"基于〈中华气功史陈列馆〉科普教育基地为核心的〈中医气功文化平台〉建设"(项目编号: ZY3-WHJS-1-1010)资助。

编者

Traditional Chinese health cultivation includes a variety of body-mind exercises, which are deeply rooted in ancient Chinese philosophy and medicine.

Today, the concept of 'health initiative (an ability to achieve physical, mental and social well-being)' has become well recognized.

Traditional Chinese health cultivation exercises are attracting worldwide attention because of their unique effects in regulating the breathing, body and mind. However, there are few books in this regard, especially the classical book series. There are even fewer bilingual Chinese-English versions of these books.

Based on their previous studies, research staff at the Shanghai Qigong Research Institute compiled eight traditional and classical health cultivation exercise methods, covering their history, theoretical foundation, characteristics and key principles, illustrated movements and application. Then these contents have been translated by professional interpreters at Shanghai University of Traditional Chinese Medicine. The Chinese version was reviewed by an expert team. The English version was reviewed by Dr. Lawrence Lau at the Yo San University of Traditional Chinese Medicine.

In addition to illustrations and videos and are also available for readers, especially overseas health cultivation fans to learn.

This books series have been funded by the Three-Year Action Plan for Chinese Medicine in Shanghai (2015-2018) on Construction of Qigong Cultural Platform in the Museum of Chinese Qigong History (Program No: ZY3–WHJS–1–1010).

Compilers

目 录

Table of Contents

1 **源流**
History

5 **理论基础**
Theoretical Foundation

6 脏腑学说与气功
Zang-fu theory and Qigong

9 **特色与要领**
Characteristics and Essential Principles

10 功法特色
Characteristics of *Song Rou Gong*

10 简单易学，舒适安全
Safe, comfortable and easy-to learn

10 动作缓慢，均匀连贯
Slow, even and continuous movements

11 动中求静，动静结合
Stillness in motion and motion in stillness

11 意气相随，形神合一
Unity of mind-qi and body-mind

12 注意"内劲"的锻炼
Exercise of internal strength

13 功法要领
Essential Principles of *Song Rou Gong*

13 心静体松，无为自然
Keep a relaxed body and tranquil mind

14 准确活泼，动作柔和
Keep an accurate posture and soft movements

15 呼吸自然，如蚕吐丝
Keep natural breathing like silkworms spinning silk

15　练养相兼，循序渐进
Balance physical exercise and rest

16　引气归原，气沉丹田
Return qi to its origin and let qi sink to Dantian

19　**功法操作**
Movements of *Song Rou Gong*

20　基础操作
Basic Movements

20　基本手型
Basic hand postures

22　基本步型
Basic stances

24　基本身型
Basic standing postures

25　具体操作
Individual Movements

25　预备势　松静站立
Preparation posture　Stand in relaxation and tranquil

28　第一势　展体舒气
Movement # 1　Stretch the body to soothe qi

32　第二势　开阔胸怀
Movement # 2　Opening up the chest

36　第三势　抱球托天
Movement # 3　Hold a balloon to lift the sky

40　第四势　转体探掌
Movement # 4　Turn the body to push the palms

45　第五势　拗身回望
Movement # 5　Turn the body to look back

51　第六势　双手举鼎
Movement # 6　Lift the tripod with both hands

56 第七势　左右侧弯
Movement # 7　Bend to left and right

62 第八势　按摩丹田
Movement # 8　Massage Dantian

65 **应用**
Application

66 功理
Mechanism

66 形体导引
Dao Yin movements of the body

68 意念导引
Dao Yin of the intent

69 呼吸导引
Dao Yin of breathing

71 作用
Functions

77 **经络图**
The Meridian Charts

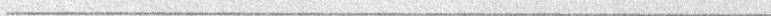

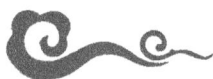

松 柔 功 • *Song Rou Gong* (Soft and Relaxed Exercise)

History

源流

松柔功是气功临床医疗中常用的基础导引功法之一。它来源于由太极拳演化而来的太极气功、道家内丹南派功法以及医家脊柱导引等功法。它秉承了太极拳松沉柔和的要领、道家清静自然无为的意境和医家行气活血通络的宗旨，通过形、意、气的导引，重点锻炼脊柱、四肢和心、肝、脾、肺、肾等脏腑功能，其中有肢体运动导引而放松身心的，有意念引导而放松入静的，有通过伸筋拔骨而先紧后松的，还有形意合一而蕴含内劲等各种方法。在功法习练中要求静心用意，呼吸自然，中正安舒，柔和缓慢，动作弧形，圆活完整，轻灵沉着，刚柔相济，慢慢由浅入深达到身心合一的功法境界。

As a common introductory *Dao Yin* exercise in clinical qigong treatment, *Song Rou Gong* derives from Taiji Quan, southern branch of internal alchemy tradition and *Dao Yin* exercise of the spine. As a result, it contains essential principles of relaxation, softness and focus on the lower body in Taiji, insight of inaction and naturalness in Daoism and circulating qi and blood in medicine. Through *Dao Yin* exercise of the body, mind and qi, *Song Rou Gong* mainly works on the spine, four limbs and functions of the heart, liver, spleen, lung and kidney. This exercise uses body movements to relax the body and mind, uses intent to guide relaxation and tranquility and combines tendon stretching with internal strength. During exercise of *Song Rou Gong*, one needs to concentrate the mind, breathe naturally, keep the body upright and conduct soft, slow movements. Over time, one can achieve a light and agile upper body, a solid lower body and body-mind unity.

随着现代社会文明的发展，我们的物质条件越来越好，但是我们所受到的社会压力也越来越大，如学习、工作、生活等等，所以消耗了我们更多的生命精华(精、气、神)，使得我们的身体更容易退变老化，心理更容易耗散疲惫，因此身心会百病丛生。而习练养生气功如本套松柔功可帮助我们扭转这种趋势，使我们的身体消除紧张僵硬，恢复柔韧有力；使我们的心理消除紧张执着，恢复平和喜悦，同时促进精气神逐渐恢复，对各种身心疾病如冠心病、老慢支、慢性胃炎、慢性肾炎、便秘、失眠、骨关节退行性病变、性功能障碍、焦虑症、抑郁症等等均有较好的效果。

Along with the advance of the society, we tend to have more and more stresses in our study, work and life. These stresses consume our essence, qi and spirit and make us vulnerable to psychological fatigue and age-related degeneration. Health qigong including *Song Rou Gong* can help to relax our body and mind and restore our essence, qi and spirit. In addition, it can benefit people with coronary artery disease, chronic bronchitis, chronic gastritis, chronic nephritis, constipation, insomnia, degenerative osteoarthritis, sexual dysfunction, anxiety and depression.

导引，是中国传统祛病养生的重要方法之一。"导"古代作疏通、宣导解。"引"有伸展，引使之意。《灵枢·官能》上说："理血气而调诸逆顺，察阴阳而兼诸方，缓节柔筋而心和调者，可使导引行气。"本功法是上海市气功研究所传统经典功法之一，它是以形体导引为基础，以良性意念调节为主导，以与形体意念导引相结合的自然轻柔的呼吸为推动力的一套整体健身运动，在心理上可以调节改善人的紧张不安情绪与不良思维，使人心情舒畅、朝气蓬勃、充满活力；在生理上可进行整体性的自我调节，有效地促进血液循环，增强脏腑功能，提高人体的适应能力和抵抗疾病的能力，从而达到健身强体、防治疾病的目的。通过习练本功法可以达到"松入筋、柔入骨"的形神合一的气功妙境。

Dao Yin is one of the leading methods in traditional health cultivation. The first word *Dao* means to dredge and guide and the second word *Yin* means to stretch and pull. The *Ling Shu Guan Neng Pian* (chapter 73 of the Spiritual Pivot) states, '... can be treated with acupuncture harmonize qi and blood and observe the abundance or insufficiency of yin and yang; those with flexible joint movements and a peaceful mind can be treated with *Dao Yin* (guiding and stretching) to circulate qi'. *Song Rou Gong* in this text is one of the classical exercises developed by Shanghai Research Institute. It is based on *Dao Yin* movements of the body, guided by positive mental intent and combined with natural breathing. Mentally, it can relieve stress, uneasiness and negative thinking, and obtain a happy mood and vitality. Physically, it can circulate blood, strengthen functions of zang-fu organs, increase adaptability and disease-defending capability of the body and achieve health. Through persistent exercise, one can achieve the amazing qigong state of body-mind unity — *relaxation into your tendons and softness into your bones.*

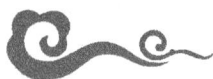

松 柔 功 • *Song Rou Gong* (Soft and Relaxed Exercise)

Theoretical Foundation

理论基础

脏腑学说与气功

Zang-fu theory and Qigong

脏腑学说是传统中医理论的重要内容，也是气功理论的重要组成部分。脏腑学说又称藏象学说，是通过观察人体外在现象、征象，来研究人体内在脏腑的生理功能、病理变化及其相互关系的学说。包括构成人体的基本结构——五脏、六腑、奇恒之腑、经络等全身组织器官的生理、病理及其相互关系；藏象学说就是建立在阴阳五行学说基础上的关于人体等级结构的模型。肝、心、脾、肺、肾五脏，配木、火、土、金、水五行，构成了互相联系制约的多体稳定系统，这也是人体稳态机制的一种模型。人体内有五脏、六腑，是人体的核心脏器，主宰着人体的生命活动。人有五官，内通五脏的外窍。肾与耳相通，肝与目相通，肺与鼻相通，心与舌相通，脾与口相通。人体的躯体有皮、肉、脉、筋、骨，也分属五脏所主管，肺主管皮毛，脾主管肌肉，心主管脉，肝主管筋，肾主管骨。五脏与六腑相配合，中医学中称为"相合"，又叫"互为表里"，脏为阴属里，腑为阳属表。以五脏为核心，配合六腑，主管五体，开窍五官，相互联系，内外沟通，形成了人的生命整体现象。

Zang-fu theory is a key part of Chinese medicine and qigong practice. Also known as *Zang Xiang* theory, Zang-fu theory studies physiology and pathology of internal organs as well as their interactions through observing external signs and manifestations. Internal organs here include five-zang organs, six-fu organs, extraordinary organs, associated tissues and meridians. *Zang Xiang* theory is based on yin-yang and five-element theory. Five-zang organs are the liver, heart, spleen, lung and kidney. They correspond to wood, fire, earth, metal and water in five-element theory. These interconnected and mutually inhibited organs constitute the homeostasis of the human body. Five-zang and six-fu organs dominate our vital activities. Five sense organs connect internally with the five zang organs: the kidney opens into the ears, the liver opens into the eyes, the lung opens into the nose, the heart opens into the tongue and the spleen opens into the mouth. The five zang organs also dominate five tissues: the lung dominates skin and skin hair, the spleen dominates muscles, the heart dominates vessels, the liver dominates tendons and the kidney dominates bones. In Chinese medicine, five-zang and six-fu organs are internal-externally connected through meridians; and five-zang organs are the core of *Zang Xiang* theory.

五脏的"脏",有"藏"的意思,就是贮藏人体的各种精气,用来维持人的生命活动。例如:心藏神,肺藏魄,肝藏魂,脾藏意,肾藏志。五脏各有职能,心脏如同国家的最高领导者,主宰全身,人的精神、意识、思维活动都是由心脏发生。心脏的功能正常,则其他脏腑就会正常发挥各自的作用。如果心脏的功能失常,则其他脏腑的功能就会受到影响,形体就会受到严重的损害。

The word *Zang* also means to store, i.e., to store essential qi to maintain vital activities. For example, the heart stores the mind, the lung stores the corporeal soul, the liver stores ethereal soul, the spleen stores intent and the kidney stores willpower. Like leadership of a country, five-zang organs dominate the body. The heart dominates mental, conscious and thinking activities. Normal functioning of the heart guarantees normal functioning of other zang organs. However, dysfunctions of the heart can affect other zang organs, severely harming the body.

气功锻炼可以协调脏腑的功能，以免出现太过或不及的状态，从而保持人体身心和谐健康。练气功通过意守丹田，使心肾相交，维持水火阴阳的动态平衡，达到涵养精气神的目的。因此练功日久，首先可见睡眠改善，精神振奋的效果。于是头晕耳鸣、失眠健忘、心悸腰酸、遗精早泄等心肾不交的症状逐步解除。意守丹田还能使心火下降温养脾土，而脾胃是向人体提供营养和能源的系统，有运化水谷精微的功能。所以练功后食欲改善，消化良好，体重平衡，是气功最明显的效验。

Qigong exercise can harmonize functions of zang-fu organs and maintain body-mind wellness. Through concentrating the mind on Dantian, qigong exercise can coordinate heart fire and kidney water, maintain dynamic yin-yang balance and nourish essence, qi and spirit. Consequently, long-time qigong practice can improve sleep quality and alleviate symptoms due to incoordination between heart fire and kidney water such as dizziness, tinnitus, insomnia, poor memory, palpitations, lumbar soreness, nocturnal emissions and premature ejaculations. In addition, focus the concentration on Dantian can reduce heart fire and warm the spleen. Since the spleen and stomach transform and transport water and grains and thus generate qi and blood, qigong practice can also improve appetite, promote digestion and benefit health.

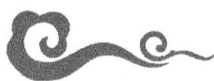

松 柔 功 • *Song Rou Gong* (Soft and Relaxed Exercise)

Characteristics and Essential Principles

特色与要领

功 法 特 色

Characteristics of *Song Rou Gong*

简单易学, 舒适安全

Safe, comfortable and easy-to learn

松柔功共有八节, 每节只有2～3个简单动作, 但又包含着柔和、舒展、优美、意气相随、形神合一的特点, 体现出气功的调身、调息、调心的特色。该功法具有安全性, 无偏差之类副作用, 易被广大中老年练功者接受和掌握。

Song Rou Gong has a total of 8 movements. Each movement contains 2-3 simple moves only; however, these moves are soft, stretching and elegant, manifesting the qigong characteristics of regulating the body, breathing and mind. In addition, these movements are safe and easy to be accepted by the middle-aged and elderly qigong fans.

动作缓慢, 均匀连贯

Slow, even and continuous movements

本功法调身以上升下降、前伸后展、左右平衡的肢体导引动作为主, 每个动作都要求做得均匀缓慢、连贯自如、轻松舒展。通过一升一降、一开一合、一左一右的起落运转等动作, 对调动全身的气机, 疏通经络、调和气血、平衡阴阳起很大作用。

Song Rou Gong mainly involves ascending, descending, extension, flexion and left-right balancing *Dao Yin* movements. Each movement needs to be even, slow and continuous. These ascending, descending, opening, closing and left-right rotation can activity qi activity, unblock meridians, harmonize qi and blood and balance yin and yang.

动中求静,动静结合
Stillness in motion and motion in stillness

本功法动中求静,肢体向上下左右运动时,都有一定的次数与程序,要配合意念和呼吸锻炼。特别要引导注意力自然集中,这实际上就是一个诱导入静的过程。这样的外动内静,还起到了调动体内"内气"运转的作用。本功法的动作以静御动,虽动犹静,形动神静。这一要求贯彻动作的始终,由松静站立而始,至拍打放松而终。

During practice of *Song Rou Gong*, upward, downward, left and right movement of the limbs needs to follow the requirements for frequency and sequence. In addition, mental intent and breathing exercise should be integrated into body movements. It's especially important to naturally concentrate the mind, which in turn regulate the flow of internal qi. *Song Rou Gong* contains stillness (mind) in motion (body movements) and motion in stillness. It starts with standing in relaxation and tranquil and ends with tapping the body.

意气相随,形神合一
Unity of mind-qi and body-mind

本功法以形导气,意气相随,上下协调,内外相合,在手足开与合、上与下的同时，心意也随之开合与上下。神为形体之帅，形为精神之载，举动轻灵，形神合一。

Song Rou Gong uses the body movements to guide qi and coordinate qi with mind while ascending, descending, opening and closing the hands and feet. Mind is the commander of body and body carries the mind, the mind and body are united as one.

注意"内劲"的锻炼
Exercise of internal strength

本功法八式的每个动作，不仅在于锻炼身体的力量，更在于通过练气和练意，来锻炼身体内部的"内力"，因此本功法也可称作是一种内功训练。在练习中动作不可僵硬，以意随形，不管是升降开合，还是左右推掌动作都要求"形、意、气"三结合，外表动，内在也随之而动，动作不是表现外力，而是显示"内劲"。

During *Song Rou Gong* exercise, each of the eight movements not only exercises the physical strength, but also exercises the internal strength through regulating qi and mind. As a result, it's important to avoid rigid movements but use mind to guide body movements and always integrate body, mind and qi in all movements (ascending, descending, opening, closing and pushing palms to left or right). In other words, these movements do not manifest external force but internal strength.

功 法 要 领
Essential Principles of *Song Rou Gong*

心静体松，无为自然
Keep a relaxed body and tranquil mind

　　心静体松是气功锻炼的基本要求，也是最根本的原则。本功法的原则要领首先要从松、静、自然入手。"松"指形体方面的放松。具体来说，就是生理状态的放松，也就是不紧张，使全身机体处在松弛、舒适状态。松是一个由浅到深、由外至内的锻炼过程，通过习练本功法使身体、呼吸、意念均慢慢进入轻松舒适的状态。"静"指思想和情绪的平稳安宁，排除杂念干扰。松与静是相辅相成的，精神上的"静"可以促使形体上的"松"，而形体上的"松"又可助于精神上的"静"，二者缺一不可。"无为自然"是指形体、呼吸、意念都要顺其自然，勿刻意追求。

　　A relaxed body and tranquil mind are essential requirement and fundamental principle to qigong practice. *Song Rou Gong* starts with *Song* (relaxation) and *Jing* (tranquility). The word *Song* means relaxation of the body, i.e., relaxation of physiological state. It takes time and practice to obtain relaxation of body, breathing and mind. The word *Jing* means a tranquil mind and emotion without distracting thoughts. Relaxation and tranquility supplement each other: mental tranquility can help body relaxation and vice versa. In addition, it's also important not to deliberately control your body, breathing and mind, just act naturally.

准确活泼，动作柔和
Keep an accurate posture and soft movements

习练本功法时，一定要保持姿势的正确，否则，就会影响练功的效果。在学习的开始阶段，正确的身形极为重要。本功法的正确姿势是：身体放松，端正自然，头顶同会阴始终保持垂直，避免挺胸、凸肚、弓背、突臀，上下、左右转动时，要保持身体松和腹实胸宽的状态，上身要灵活，下身要稳重。转动时要以腰为轴心，以腰转动来带动四肢运动。腰要保持松沉直竖，不软塌，不摇晃。骶部要沉着有力，使重心下降稳定。肩要松沉，肘要松垂，头要正直，颈项虽直而不僵硬。练功过程中始终要保持心静体松，动作要柔和舒展、上下协调、内外相合、灵活连贯。

It's important for beginners to keep an accurate posture during *Song Rou Gong* practice, because it's directly associated with the effect of exercise. An accurate posture contains a relaxed upright body and a straight line of Baihui[1] (DU 20) and Huiyin[2] (Ren 1). Chest/belly out, hollow back and lifted buttocks should be avoided. While turning the body, remember to keep the body upright, a flexible upper body and solid lower body and use the waist as an axis. In addition, it's advisable to use the rotation of the waist to move the limbs and, at the same time, keep the waist relaxed but solid. The sacral region needs to be strong and solid to stabilize the body weight. The shoulders and elbows need to be relaxed and dropped. The head needs to be upright. The neck needs to be upright but not rigid. It's essential to maintain a relaxed body, a tranquil mind

---

1. An acupuncture point located at the junction of a line connecting the apices of the ears (in the middle).

2 An acupuncture point located at the midpoint between the root of the scrotum and the anus in males, and at the midpoint between the posterior labial commissure and the anus in females.

and soft coordinated body movements during the exercise.

呼吸自然，如蚕吐丝
Keep natural breathing like silkworms spinning silk

呼吸自然指本功法锻炼过程中采用自然呼吸的方法，不刻意追求特殊的呼吸形式（如逆腹式呼吸等），以利于身心放松、心平气和及身体的协调运动。通过长期锻炼，自然呼吸会慢慢变得柔和、深长、缓慢、流畅。练习本功时充分运用良性意念，并意守手掌心、脚底心、腹部丹田、命门等部位或穴位，这样在呼吸过程中便能强化丹田之气。

Instead of special intentional breathing (such as reverse abdominal breathing), natural breathing is recommended in *Song Rou Gong* practice for body-mind relaxation and coordinated physical movements. Over time, the breathing can gradually become soft, deep, slow and even. It's also important to use positive thinking and focus the mental concentration on Laogong (PC 8), Yongquan (KI 1), Dantian and Mingmen area. This can help to strengthen qi of Dantian.

练养相兼，循序渐进
Balance physical exercise and rest

初学阶段，要讲究有动有静，动静不可偏废，练养不可脱离。初练者在练功过程中，身体会产生某些不适，如肌肉关节酸痛、动作僵硬、手脚配合不协调等等，因此需要形体的静养，不能操之过急，急于追求效果而盲目硬练，则会出现疲劳过度，对身体健康有害。只有经过一段时间的习练，肢体的动作才会越来连贯，"形神"才会越来越协调，练功的效果才会显现。练功者切忌"三天打鱼，两天晒网"，松懈、疲沓地练功是不可能获得效果的，而应一步一步地按照练功的原则和方法，并且根据自己的身体状况，持之以恒，循序渐进，力求不断提高练功质量，这样才能使自己的身心得到提升。

It's advisable for beginners to do physical exercise and have plenty of rest. During qigong practice, some beginners may experience physical discomfort such as muscle or joint pain, stiff or rigid movements and hand-foot incoordination. It's therefore necessary to get rest. Overhastiness may cause fatigue and is harmful to the body. It takes time to obtain continuity of the body movements and body-mind coordination. You'll never succeed if you 'spend three days fishing and then two days drying nets' (a Chinese proverb, referring to people who lack perseverance and don't persist on doing things). You need to practice step by step according to your own physical condition and improve your exercise quality as well as your body-mind wellness.

引气归原，气沉丹田
Return qi to its origin and let qi sink to Dantian

大凡气功练习，在练功结束前都必须进行"收功"收本功法也不例外。由于"收功"对练功是否取得成效有一定关系，所以历代气功家对"收功"极为重视，并创编了不少收功法。所有收功法都有一个共同的特点，即把全身的"气息"引导回归到腹部"丹田"处，在气功锻炼中称作"引气归元"，或称为"气息归根"。本功法第八节按摩丹田，首先用意念把全身的"气息"缓慢地引导到腹部丹田，接着再做按摩功，按顺时针和逆时针方向，先后以丹田为中心沿上下左右方向摩腹各9次，这样有助于达到上体虚灵、下体充实之目的。

Most qigong practices need to 'close' before they are concluded, and so does *Song Rou Gong*. Since 'closing' is associated with the exercise result, qigong masters of different generations highly valued 'closing' and developed many closing methods. These methods share a common feature — to return qi of the body to Dantian, known as 'return qi to its origin' in qigong exercise. Take movement # 8 (massage Dantian) for example, first use the intent to slowly guide qi to Dantian and then massage 9 times clockwise and counterclockwise respectively around Dantian, thus achieving an unweighted upper body but solid lower body.

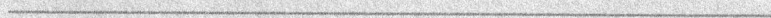

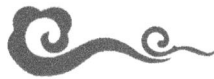

松 柔 功 • *Song Rou Gong* (Soft and Relaxed Exercise)

Movements of *Song Rou Gong*

功法操作

基 础 操 作

Basic Movements

本功法的基础动作——手型、步型、身型：

Basic movements of *Song Rou Gong* are hand postures, stances and standing postures.

基本手型

Basic hand postures

1. 自然手型

1. Natural hand posture

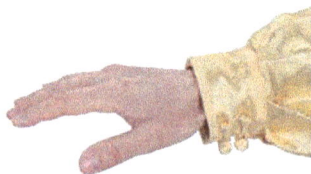

五指放松伸直、自然并拢。

Relax, extend and put all five fingers together.

手型图1　Hand posture 1

2. 抱球状手型

2. Balloon-holding posture

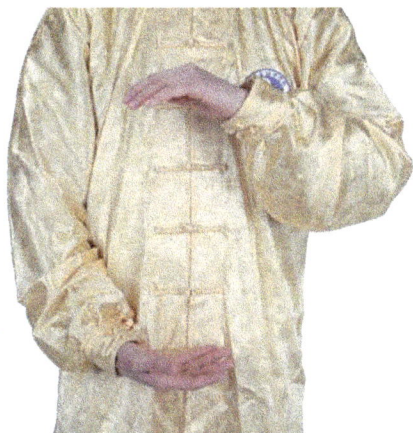

两手十指自然舒展,掌心相对,一手在上,位于膻中前,一手在下,位于丹田前,似抱一气球。

Stretch the fingers, let the palms facing each other, place one hand in front of Danzhong (Ren 17) and the other hand in front of Dantian, and pretend to hold an inflated balloon.

手型图2　Hand posture 2

3. 立掌、推掌型

3. Standing or pushing palm

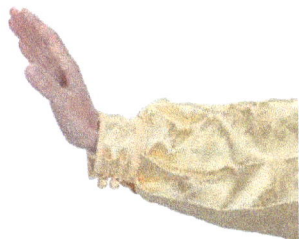

两手竖掌,五指放松伸直、自然并拢,平行向前或向两侧推掌。

With standing palms, relax, extend and put all five fingers together, push the palm forward or to both sides in parallel.

手型图3　Hand posture 3

基本步型
Basic stances

1. 开立步型

1. Open stance (*Kai Li Bu*)

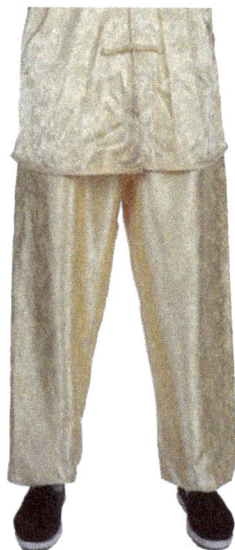

步型图 1   Stance 1

两脚分开，两脚外侧与肩同宽，两膝关节自然伸直。

Separate the feet to make lateral sides of the feet at shoulder-width apart and naturally extend the knee joints.

2. 虚步型

2. Empty (unweighted) stance (*Xu Bu*)

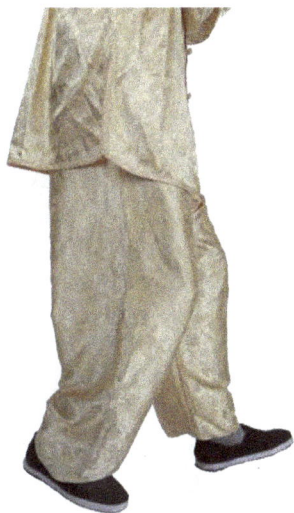

分为左虚步型与右虚步型。左虚步型身体的重心位于右腿,左腿位于身前半步,脚跟着地,脚尖上翘。

右虚步型与左虚步型相同,唯方向相反。

Left unweighted stance places the body weight on the right (back) leg. The left leg is half a step forward with the heel touching the floor and toes pointing up.

Right unweighted stance: same stance in an opposite direction.

步型图 2　Stance 2

3. 弓步型

3. Bow stance (*Gong Bu*)

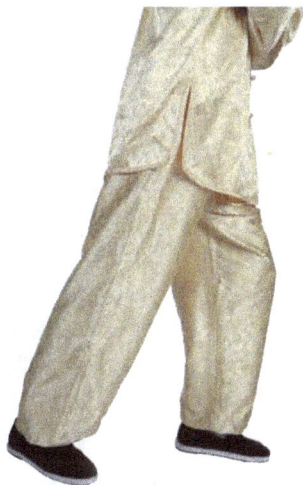

分为左弓步型和右弓步型。左弓步型左腿在身前半步屈曲,右腿向后伸直,重心位于两腿中间,右弓步型与左弓步型相同,唯方向相反。

Left bow stance: The left leg is half a step forward and bent at the knee, the back right leg straight, and the body weight is placed between the two legs .

Right bow stance: Same stance in an opposite direction.

步型图 3　Stance 3

基本身形
Basic standing postures

1. 自然站立型
1. Natural standing

　　两脚分开与肩等宽，两手自然下垂，人体重心在两脚之间，身体一定要站稳，做到"站如松"。

　　Separate the feet at shoulder-width apart, drop the hands to the sides, place the body weight between the feet, and keep the body upright like a pine tree.

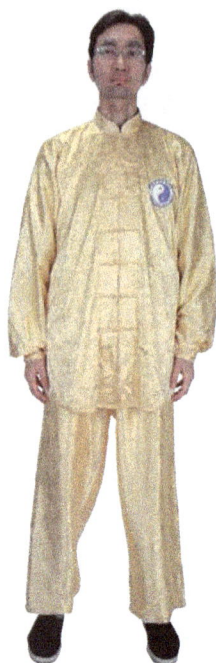

身型图1　Standing posture 1

2. 高位马步站桩型
2. High-position horse stance standing

　　两脚分开站立，两膝微屈，膝面不超过脚尖，两脚掌着地，脚尖朝正前方，身正肩平，松肩收腹，形似骑马的姿势。

　　Separate the feet, slightly bend the knees and do not let the knees go past the toes, with the soles toughing the floor and toes pointing straight forward. Keep the body upright, square the shoulders, chest forward, belly tucked in and make a horse-riding posture .

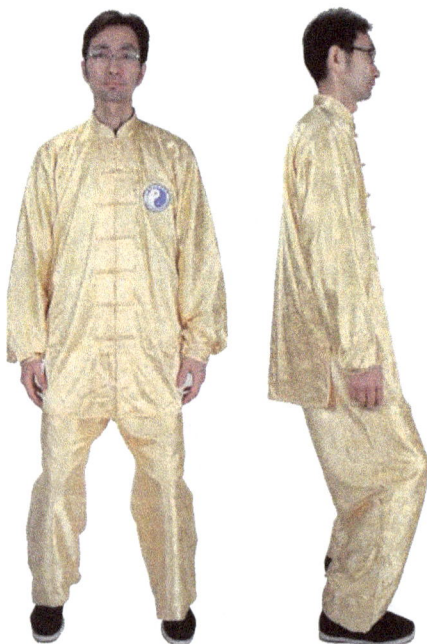

正面　　　　　　　　侧面

身型图2　Standing posture 2

具 体 操 作
Individual Movements

预备势　松静站立
Preparation posture　Stand in relaxation and tranquil

1. 调身

1. Regulating the body

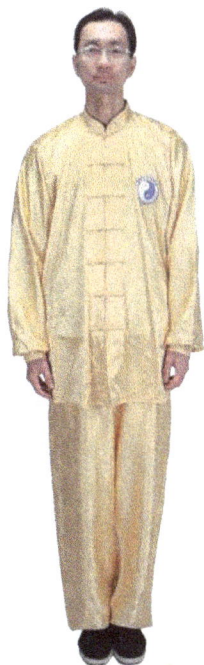

松静站立, 双脚并拢, 双目平视。

Stand in relaxation and tranquil, put the feet together and look straight ahead.

图 0-1　Fig 0-1

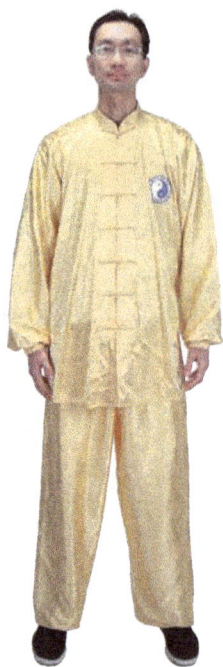

重心右移，左脚抬起向左侧分开站立，然后将重心移至两腿之间，两臂下垂。

Shift the body weight to the right, lift the left foot to the left, then shift the body weight to the area between the feet and naturally drop the arms to the sides.

图 0-2　Fig 0-2

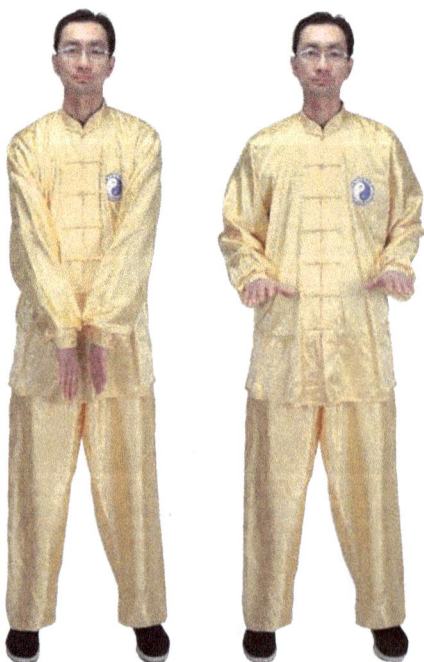

两手经体前上提，同时向两侧划圆，掌心向下（图 0-3、图 0-4）。

Lift the hands from the sides, draw circles towards the sides and make the palms downward. (Fig 0-3, Fig 0-4)

图 0-3　Fig 0-3　　　　图 0-4　Fig 0-4

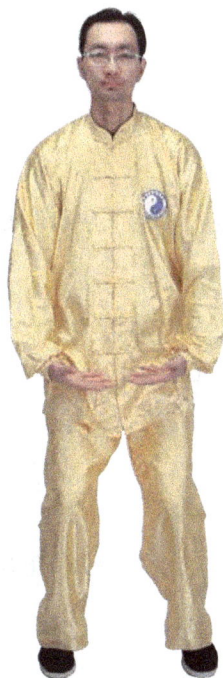

图 0-5　Fig 0-5

两手翻掌转至小腹前，同时屈膝半坐成高位桩，两掌心向上，十指相对。全身放松，两眼平视。

Turn the palms to the front of the lower abdomen, bend at the knee to make a high-position *Zhan Zhuang*, make the palms upward, and let the fingers of the hands facing each other. Relax the body and look straight ahead.

2. 调息

2. Regulating the breathing

自然呼吸。

Breath naturally.

3. 调心

3. Regulating the mind

两耳细听自己的呼吸声或凝听其他有节律的声响,诱导入静。心平气和,静立放松。

Listen carefully to one's own breathing or rhythmic sounds, keep a peaceful mind and stand in relaxation and tranquil

[操作提示]

身体要放松,精神安静,自然站立,十指相对似托物于小腹前。

呼吸自然、徐缓。鼻吸鼻呼。静立一会儿,准备练功。

[Tips]

Relax the body, have a peaceful mind, stand naturally, place the hands in front of the lower abdomen, and let the fingers of the hands facing each other.

Breathe slowly and naturally with the nose. Stay still for 30 seconds.

第一势　展体舒气

Movement # 1　Stretch the body to soothe qi

1. 调身

1. Regulating the body

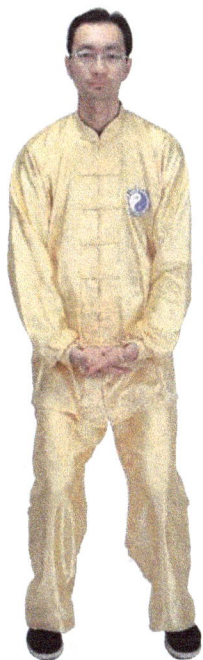

图 1-1　Fig 1-1

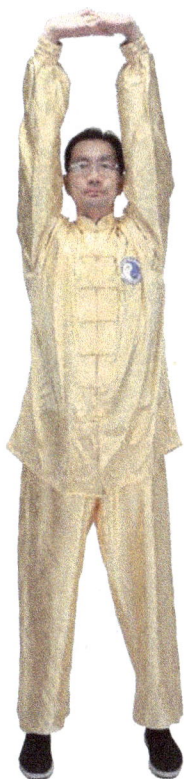

接预备势，两手在小腹前交叉，沿腹前上升至胸前，翻掌向上升过头顶，两臂伸直，掌心朝上，双目平视前方（图1-1、图1-2）。

Further to the preparation posture, cross the hands in front of the abdomen, lift the hands to the level of the chest, turn the palms and lift above the top of the head, extend the arms, make the palms upward and look straight ahead. (Fig 1-1, Fig 1-2)

图 1-2　Fig 1-2

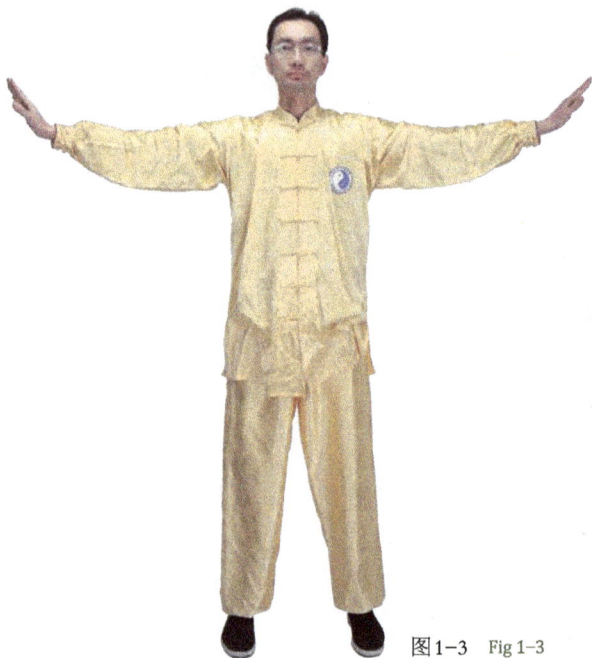

图 1-3　Fig 1-3

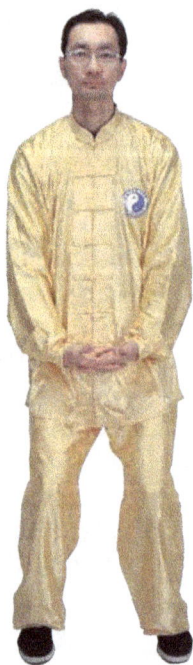

身体保持正直，把交
叉的双手自然分开，两掌
分别向左右两侧下落至两
大腿前，十指交叉置于小
腹前，掌心朝上，屈膝半坐
（图 1-3、图 1-4）。

Keep the body upright,
separate the crossed hands,
drop the palms from both sides
down to the front of the thighs,
cross fingers in front of the
lower abdomen, make the palms
upward, bend at the knees and
perform a half sitting position.
(Fig 1-3, Fig 1-4)

图 1-4　Fig 1-4

如此一起一落、一开一合，反复练习6次。

Repeat 6 times of ascending, descending, opening and closing.

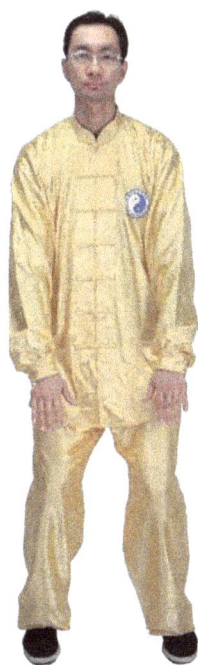

结束时，呈屈膝下蹲，两手落于大腿前，掌心向内。

Conclusion: Bend at the knees to squat down, drop the hands to the front of the thighs and make the palms inward.

图1-5 Fig 1-5

2. 调息
2. Regulating the breathing

自然呼吸。

Natural breathing.

3. 调心

3. Regulating the mind

两掌上托时意念手顶天,脚立地,排除杂念,心情保持轻松愉快。

Imagine supporting the sky with the hands and stand on the earth with the feet while lifting the palms, remove distracting thoughts and keep a relaxed and happy mind.

［操作提示］

双手上举时,全身尽量伸直,充分伸展脊柱,勿使两脚跟离地。双手下落时,全身放松,屈膝微蹲。

呼吸自然,两手上提为吸气,两手下落为呼气。

[Tips]

Straighten up the body, especially the spine while lifting the hands. Keep the heels on the floor. Relax the body, bend at the knees and slightly squat down while dropping the hands.

Breathe naturally: inhale while lifting the hands and exhale while dropping the hands.

第二势　开阔胸怀

Movement # 2 Opening up the chest

----

1. 调身

1. Regulating the body

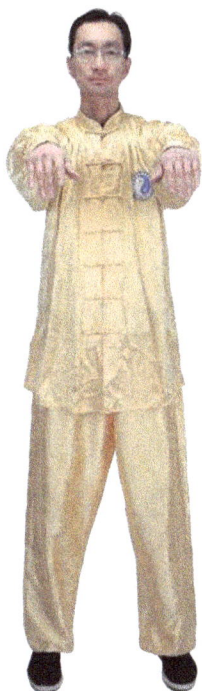

接上势，两手掌心向
下，如太极起势，两臂向
前上提至胸前，两膝逐渐
伸直。

Further to the last movement,
make the palms downward like
the starting posture of Taiji.

图2-1　Fig 2-1

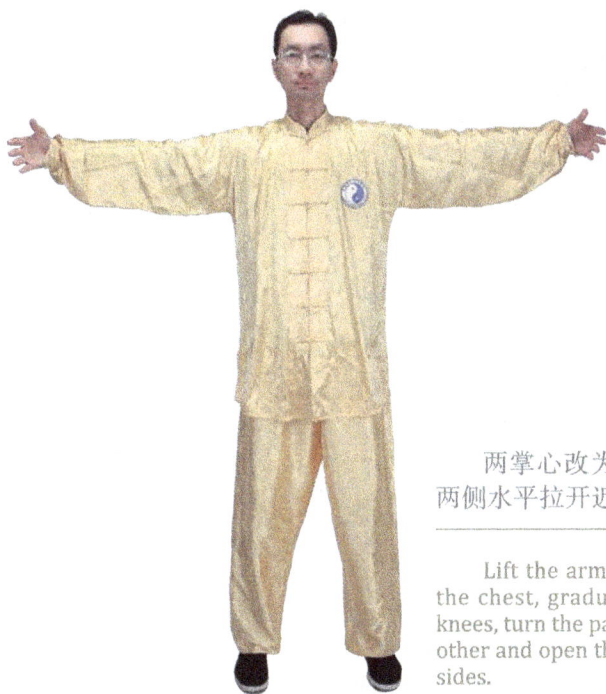

两掌心改为自然相对，向
两侧水平拉开近"一"字形。

Lift the arms to the level of
the chest, gradually extend the
knees, turn the palms to face each
other and open the palms to both
sides.

图2-2　Fig 2-2

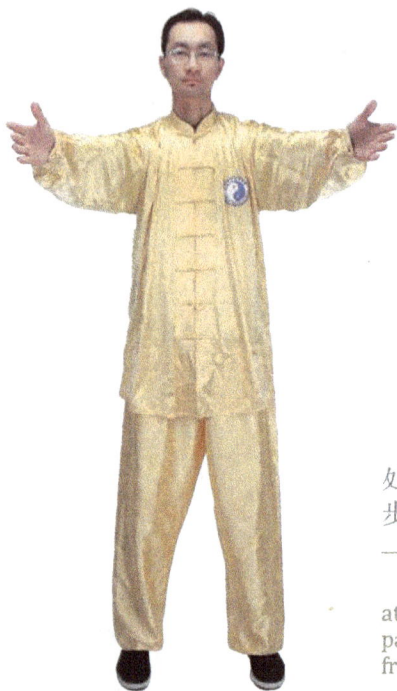

两臂向胸前相合至与肩同宽处，转为掌心向下，两臂下落，逐步屈膝，身体亦随之下降。

Close the arms towards the chest at shoulder-width distance, turn the palms downward, drop the arms to the front of the thighs and lower the body.

图2-3　Fig 2-3

如此一升一举，一开一合，反复习练6次。

Repeat 6 times of ascending, descending, opening and closing.

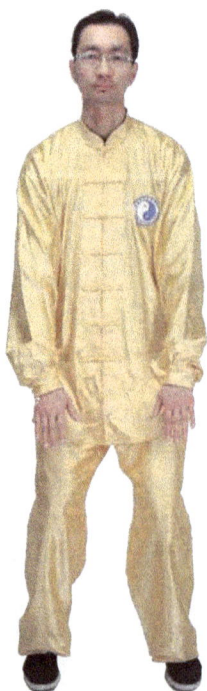

结束时，呈屈膝下蹲，两手落于大腿前，掌心向内。

Conclusion: Bend at the knees to squat down, drop the hands to the front of the thighs and make the palms inward.

图2-4　Fig 2-4

2. 调息

2. Regulating the breathing

自然呼吸，功法熟练后可配合功法动作升降开合。

Natural breathing at first; over time, ascending, descending, opening and closing can be combined with *Dao Yin* movements.

3. 调心

3. Regulating the mind

意想站在高山上，胸怀开阔，目光平视，意念始终置于两手心和十个手指间，气感绵绵不断。

Imagine standing on a high mountain with an open heart. Look straight ahead, place mental focus on the palms and spaces between fingers, and experience the uninterrupted qi sensation.

［操作提示］
两臂下落时，松腰坠髋、沉肩垂肘。
两臂提升扩展时自然吸气，合拢下降时自然呼气。

[Tips]
Relax the waist and shoulders and drop the hips and elbows while dropping the arms.

Breathe in naturally while lifting and opening up the arms and breathe out naturally while closing and dropping the arms.

第三势　抱球托天

Movement # 3 Hold a balloon to lift the sky

....

1. 调身

1. Regulating the body

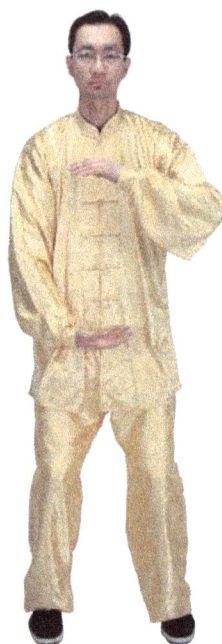

图3-1　Fig 3-1

接上势,两手从体侧提升并移至胸腹前,左手在上,右手在下,呈抱球手型,两膝微屈。

Further to the last movement, lift the hands from both sides of the body to the level of the abdomen and chest, make the balloon-holding posture with the left hand on top and right hand down, and slightly bend at the knees .

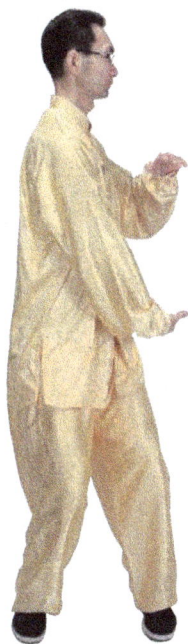

向左转腰，左手上，右手下。

Turn the waist to the left and place the left hand on top and right hand down.

图3–2　Fig 3–2

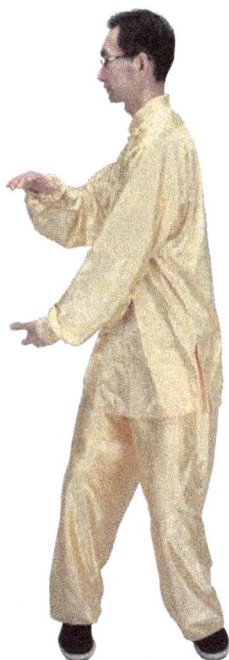

然后交换为右手上、左手下，呈抱球手型，向右转腰。再交换为左手上，右手下，呈抱球手型，向左转腰。

Then change the position of the hands (right hand on top and left hand down) to hold a balloon and turn the waist to the right. Then re-change the position of the hands (left hand on top and right hand down) to hold a balloon and turn the waist to the left.

图3–3　Fig 3–3

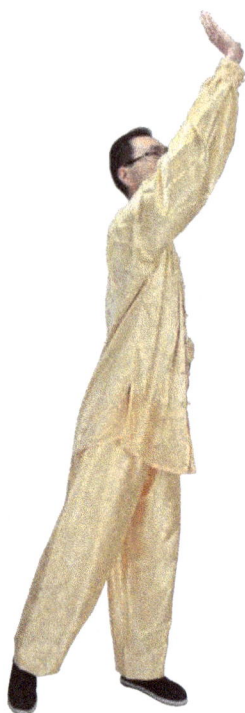

左手下按,置于左腰,全身重心移至左腿,右手托起至胸前,转掌向上,经右额前向上托掌,两眼始终注视右手前上方。

右手转掌心向下,从左上方往下降至胸前,左手从左腰至腹前,右手在上,左手在下,两掌心相对,呈抱球状手型。

Press with the left hand and place the left hand on the left side of the waist, shift the body weight to the left leg and lift the right hand to the front of the chest. Turn the palms upward and lift the palms along the front of the right forehead, and focus the eyes on the anterior and superior part of the right hand.

Turn the right palm downward and lower the right palm to the front of the chest. Lower the left hand from left side of the waist to the front of the abdomen and make the balloon-holding posture with the right hand on top and left hand down.

图 3-4　Fig 3-4

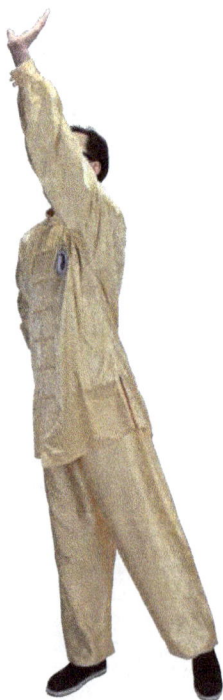

以上为左势。然后做右势,动作相同,唯方向相反。

Then turn to the waist to the right and perform the same procedure in an opposite direction.

图 3-5　Fig 3-5

左右势各做3次。

Repeat 3 times on each side.

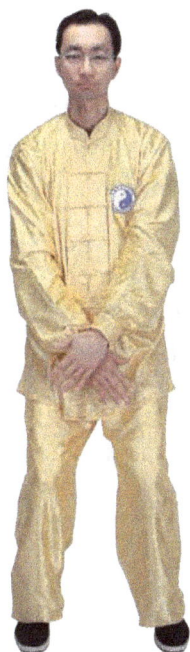

结束时，呈屈膝下蹲，双手掌心向内，
自然回落于大腿前。

Conclusion: Bend at the knees to squat
down, drop the hands to the front of the thighs
and make the palms inward.

图3-6　Fig 3-6

2. 调息

2. Regulating the breathing

自然呼吸。

Natural breathing.

3. 调心

3. Regulating the mind

意想两掌之间抱一气球，并随着手的运动而运行。

Place the mental focus on holding an inflated balloon and moving with the hand.

［操作提示］

马步高位站桩与转腰抱球时动作要协调一致。

托掌向上时，重心落于左腿或右腿之上；抱球时，身体略蹲，膝微屈。

[Tips]

A horse-stance high-position *Zhan Zhuang* needs to coordinate with turning the waist to hold a balloon.

Place the body weight on the left or right leg while lifting the palms; slightly bend at the knees and squat down while holding an inflated balloon.

第四势　转体探掌

Movement # 4 Turn the body to push the palms

1. 调身

1. Regulating the body

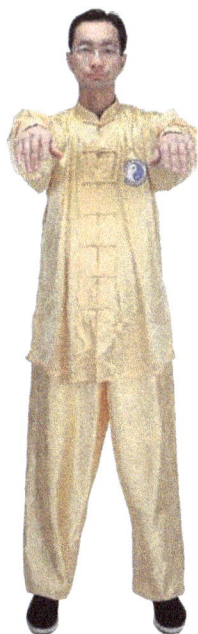

接上势，双手伸直上提与肩平，掌心向下，五指自然略分开。

Further to the last movement, extend and lift the hands to the level of the shoulders, turn the palms downward and slightly separate the five fingers.

图4-1　Fig 4-1

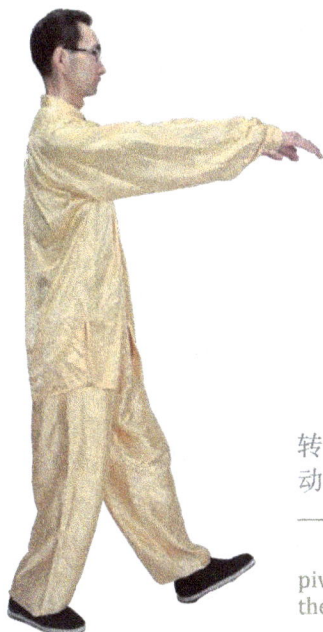

以左脚跟及右脚尖为支点，同时向左转90°，向前平伸的双手随身体向左转动，视线紧随双手。

Using the left heel and right tiptoe as the pivot, turn 90° to the left, turn the hands to the left and focus the eyes on the hands.

图4-2　Fig 4-2

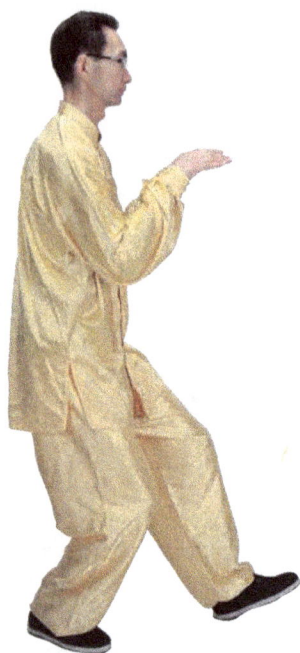

重心移至右脚,左腿伸直,左脚尖翘起,屈肘,双手向胸前收回竖掌,掌心朝前,目视前方。

Shift the body weight to the right leg, extend the left leg, curl the left tiptoe up, flex the elbows, retract the hands to the front of the chest, turn palms forward and look straight ahead.

图4-3　Fig 4-3

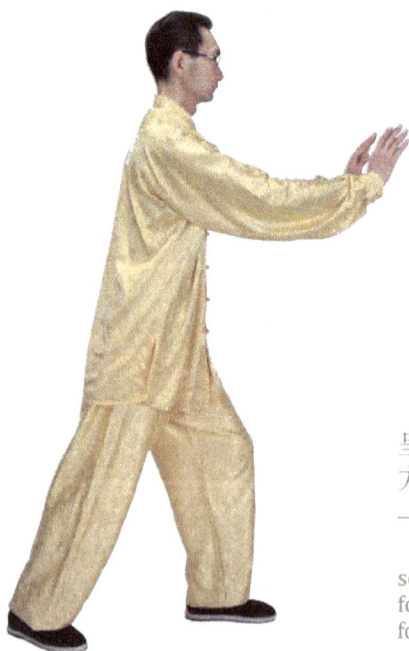

左脚掌着地,重心移至左脚呈左弓步,两掌向前推出,目视前方。

Touch the floor with the left sole, shift the body weight to the left foot (left bow step), push the palms forward and look straight ahead.

图4-4　Fig 4-4

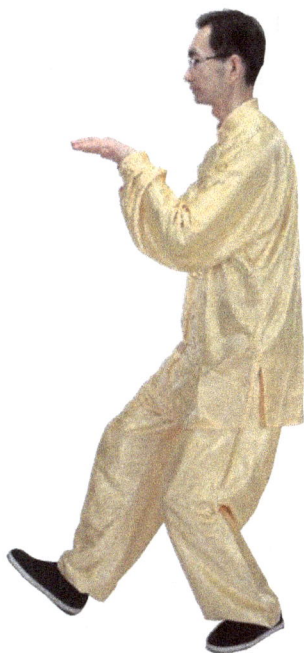

重心后移至右脚，左脚掌内
扣，重心移至左脚，身体以左脚跟
为轴向右旋转180°，两臂平行，掌
心向下，随身体向右转动。然后
右腿伸直，右脚尖翘起，屈肘，两手
向胸前收回竖掌，掌心朝前，目视
前方。

Shift the body weight to the
right foot, curl the left sole inward,
then shift the body weight to the
left foot and use the left heel as an
axis to turn 180° to the right. Make
the palms downward and turn the
paralleled arms to the right. Extend
the right leg, curl the right tiptoe up,
flex the elbows, retract the hands
to the front of the chest, turn palms
forward and look straight ahead.

图 4-5　　Fig 4-5

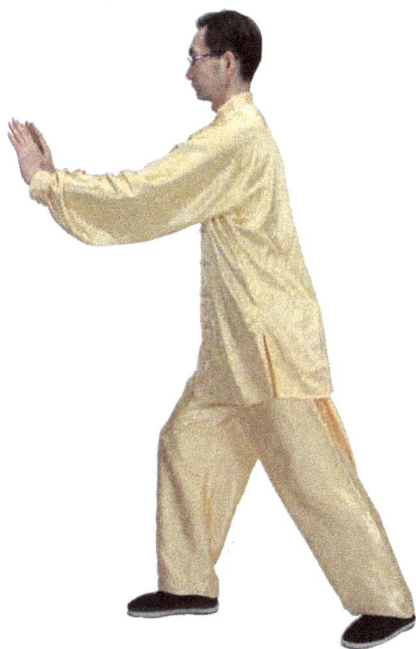

右脚掌着地，重心移至右脚，
呈右弓步，两掌向前推出。

Touch the floor with the right
sole, shift the body weight to the
right foot (right bow step), push the
palms forward and look straight
ahead.

图 4-6　　Fig 4-6

以上动作左右各习练3次。

Repeat 3 times on each side.

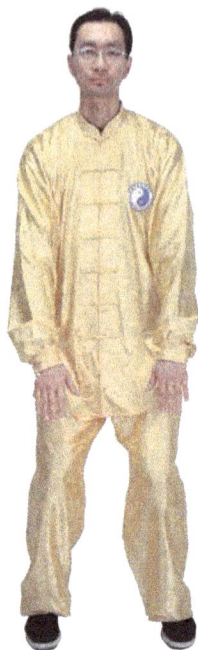

　　结束时，身体转向正前方，双手背与肩平，双目平视。然后，屈膝下蹲，两手下按，掌心向内，落于大腿前。

　　Conclusion: Turn the body straight ahead, make the dorsa of the hands at the same level of the shoulder, and look straight ahead. Conclusion: Bend at the knees to squat down, drop the hands to the front of the thighs and make the palms inward.

图 4-7　Fig 4-7

2. 调息
2. Regulating the breathing

　　自然呼吸，熟练后配合功法收掌时吸气，推掌时呼气。

　　Natural breathing at first; over time, combine inhalation while retracting the palms and exhalation while pushing the palms.

3. 调心
3. Regulating the mind

重心前移推掌时，意想两掌如推小山，注意内劲的运用。

Imagine pushing a small hill while shifting the body weight to push the palm. Pay attention to the use of internal strength.

[操作提示]

旋转时以脚跟为轴带动身体，左转时右脚尖内扣；右转时左脚尖内扣。身体重心左右转移应通过脚跟的转动来进行，并以此带动身体旋转并与两手内收和推掌动作协调一致。

[Tips]

Use the heel as an axis to turn the body, curl the right tiptoe inward while turning to the left and vice versa. Turn the heel to shift the body weight to the left or right, further to turn the body and coordinate with closing the hands and pushing the palm.

第五势　拗身回望

Movement # 5 Turn the body to look back

1. 调身

1. Regulating the body

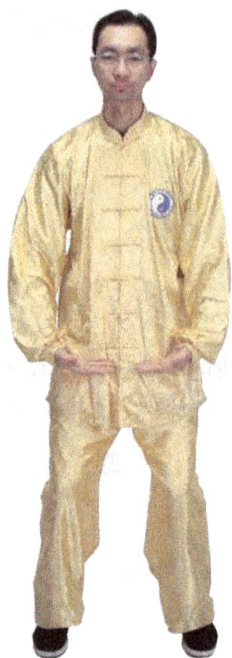

接上势，两手翻掌。

Further to the last movement, turn the palms upward.

图 5–1　Fig 5–1

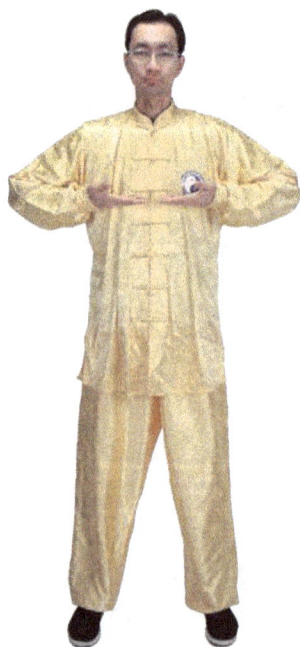

掌心向上提至胸前。

Lift the palms to the front of the chest.

图 5–2　Fig 5–2

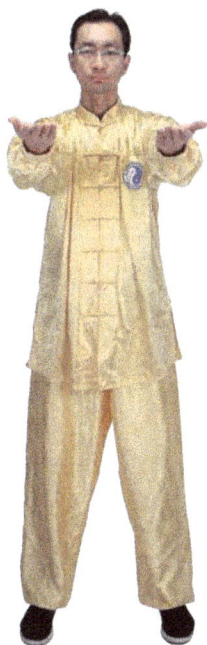

双臂向前平伸，双目平视。

Extend the arms forward and look
straight ahead.

图 5-3   Fig 5-3

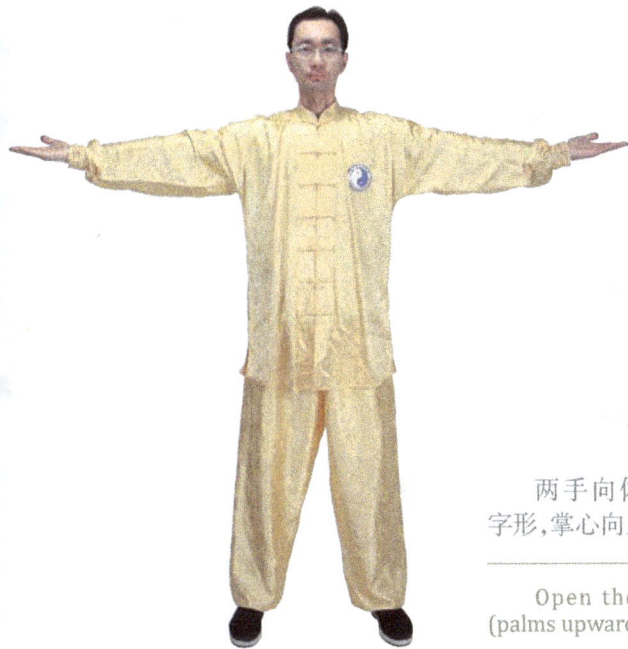

两手向体侧水平拉开呈"一"
字形，掌心向上。

Open the hands to both sides
(palms upward).

图 5-4   Fig 5-4

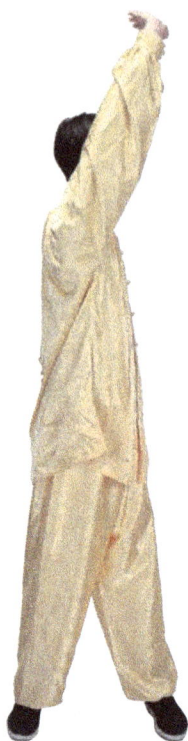

两臂随身体向左侧旋转，同时旋掌。身体逐步转向左后侧，眼看后下方，同时右手上托，高于头顶，左手背置于腰后命门处，两掌心均向外，手臂稍稍弯曲。

Turn the body and arms to the left and rotate the palm. Gradually turn the body to left rear, look backward and downward and lift the right hand above the top of the head. Place the dorsum of the left hand on the Mingmen area, turn the palms outward and slightly flex the arms.

图5—5　Fig 5-5

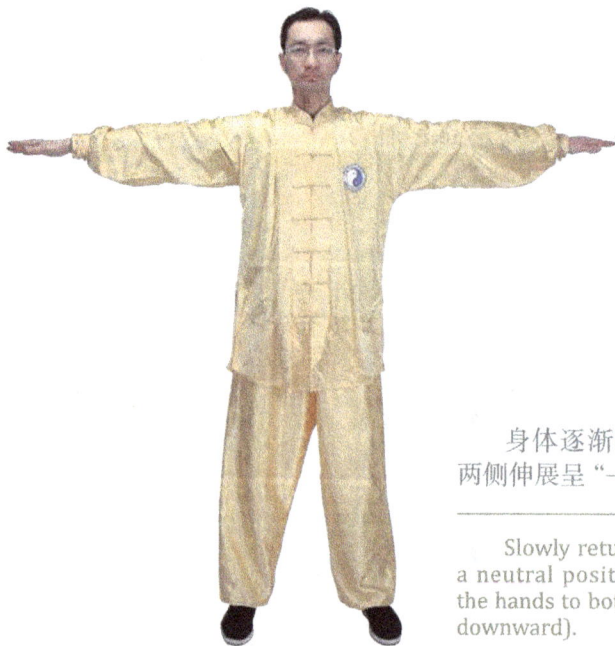

身体逐渐转正，两手向两侧伸展呈"一"字形。

Slowly return the body to a neutral position and open the hands to both sides (palms downward).

图5—6　Fig 5-6

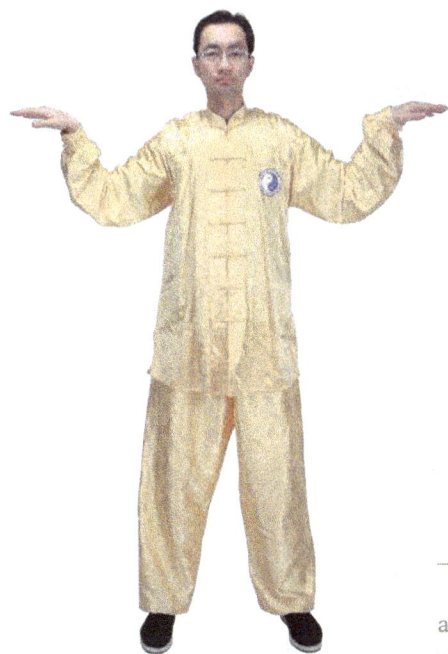

掌心向下，两臂曲肘收手。

Slightly bend at the elbows
and close the hands.

图5-7　Fig 5-7

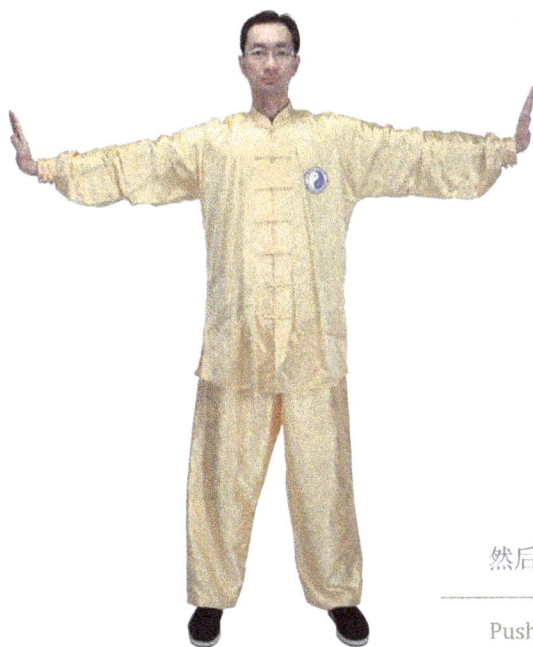

然后向外推掌。

Push the palms out .

图5-8　Fig 5-8

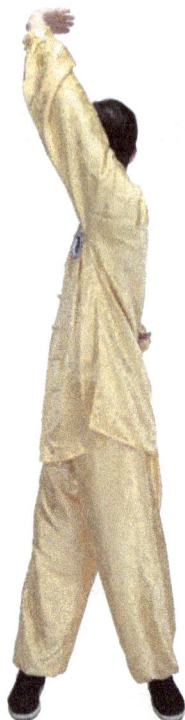

双手逐渐下落至小腹处，两膝微屈。

Slowly drop the hands down to the lower abdomen and slightly bend at the knees.

图5-9　Fig 5-9

以上是左势。右势动作与左势相同,唯方向相反。

Perform the same procedure to the right side.

左右势各习练3次。

Repeat 3 times on each side.

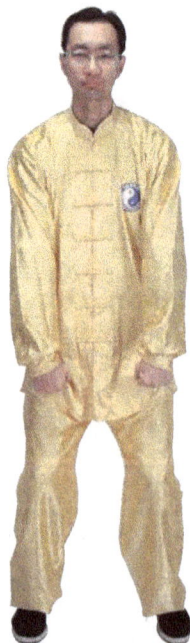

结束时,身体转向正前方,双手背与肩平,双目平视。然后,屈膝下蹲,两手下按,掌心向内,落于大腿前。

Conclusion: Turn the body to a neutral position, place the dorsa of the hands to the level of the shoulder and look ahead. Bend at the knees to squat down, drop the hands to the front of the thighs and make the palms inward.

图5-10　Fig 5-10

2. 调息

2. Regulating the breathing

自然呼吸。

Natural breathing.

3. 调心

3. Regulating the mind

内心平静，意识专注于动作上。

Keep a tranquil mind and focus the mental concentration on movements.

[操作提示]

伸展动作要以舒适为度，肩、腰、胯要放松，两膝要伸直，两脚固定不动。

[Tips]

Stretching and extension should be within the comfort zone, relax the shoulders, waist and hips. Extend the knees and do not move the feet.

第六势　双手举鼎

Movement # 6 Lift the tripod with both hands

1. 调身

1. Regulating the body

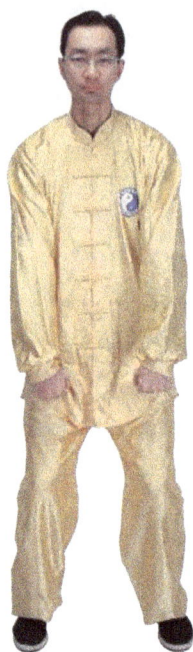

接上势，两手虚握拳，由胯前提至平腰部，两腿自然伸直，脚跟着地，气沉丹田。

Further to the last movement, make a half clench of the fists and lift the fists from the hips to the waist, extend the legs, touch the floor with the heels and let qi sink down to Dantian .

图6-1　Fig 6-1

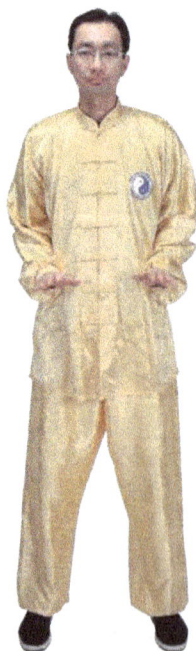

松拳，两手下按，气沉涌泉，两腿下蹲，膝面不超过足尖。

Release the fists, press down with both hands, let qi sink to Yongquan (KI 1)[1], squat down and do not let the knees go past the toes .

图6-2　Fig 6-2

---

1. An acupuncture point located on the sole, in the depression appearing on the anterior part of the sole when the foot is in the plantar flexion, approximately at the junction of the anterior third and posterior two thirds of the line connecting the base of the 2nd and 3rd toes and the heel.

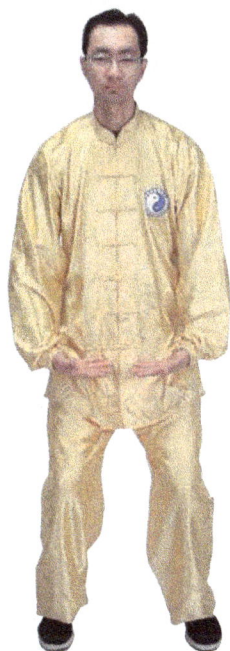

双手翻掌，置于腹前。

Turn the palms and place them in front of the abdomen.

图6-3　Fig 6-3

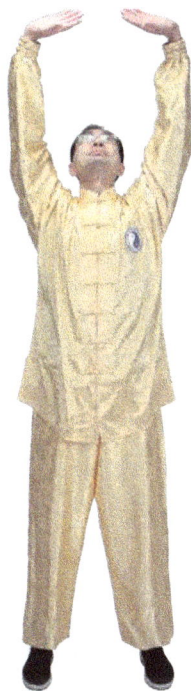

掌心向上提至膻中，再翻掌向上举过顶，两腿逐渐自然伸直，双手虎口相对，成举鼎状，脚跟着地，双目上视。

Make the palms upward and lift them to Danzhong[1] (Ren 17). Turn the palms and lift above the top of the head, slowly extend the legs, make the *Hukou* (space between the thumb and index finger) areas facing each other to lift the (imaginary) tripod, touch the floor with the heels and look upward.

图6-4　Fig 6-4

1. An acupuncture point located at the level with the 4th intercostal space, midway between the nipples.

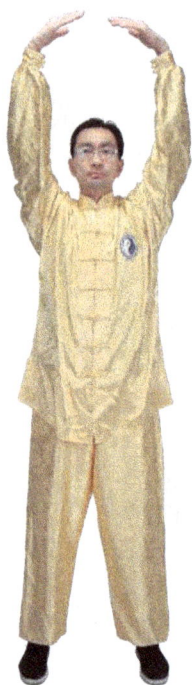

双手翻掌向下。

Turn the palms downward.

图6-5　Fig 6-5

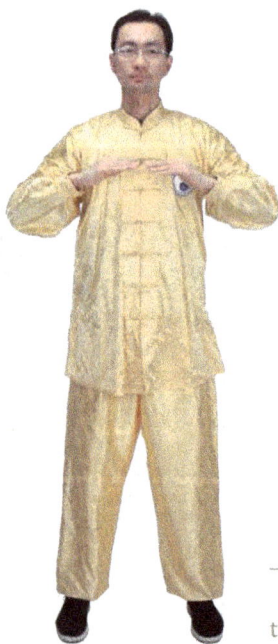

由胸前下落至大腿前，两膝微屈。

Drop them from the chest to the front of the thighs and slightly bend at the knees.

图6-6　Fig 6-6

本势动作习练6次。

Repeat 6 times.

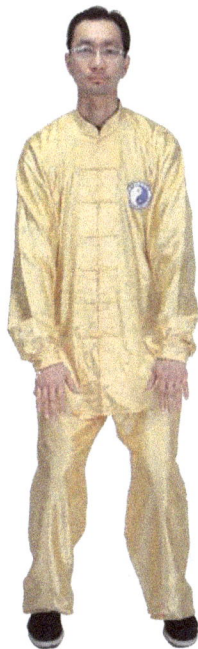

结束时，呈屈膝下蹲，两手落于大腿前，掌心向内。

Conclusion: Bend at the knees to squat down, drop the hands to the front of the thighs and make the palms inward.

图6-7　Fig 6-7

2. 调息
2. Regulating the breathing

自然呼吸。

Natural breathing.

3. 调心
3. Regulating the mind

两拳上提时意念如提重物，双掌上托时意念专注，如举鼎器，用意不用力。

Imagine lifting a heavy object while lifting the fists. Focus the mental concentration on lifting the tripod, use the intent instead of strength.

[操作提示]

[Tips]

身体及双手的动作都须垂直上下进行，不可发生偏斜。

抓拳提升时微微用劲。

Movements of the body and hands needs to be performed vertically and there should be no deviations.

Use some force to clench and lift the fists.

第七势　左右侧弯

Movement # 7 Bend to left and right

1. 调身

1. Regulating the body

接上势，身体慢慢站直，右臂伸直，从身体右侧缓缓上举，掌心向外，指尖朝上。

Further to the last movement, slowly stand upright.Extend the right arm and lift from the right side of the body slowly, making the palms outward and fingers pointing upwards.

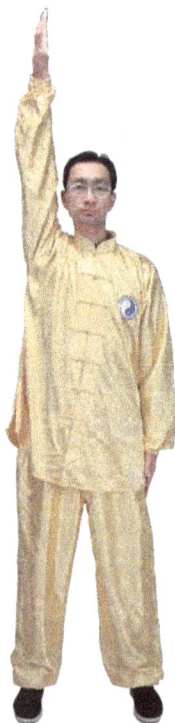

图7-1　Fig 7-1

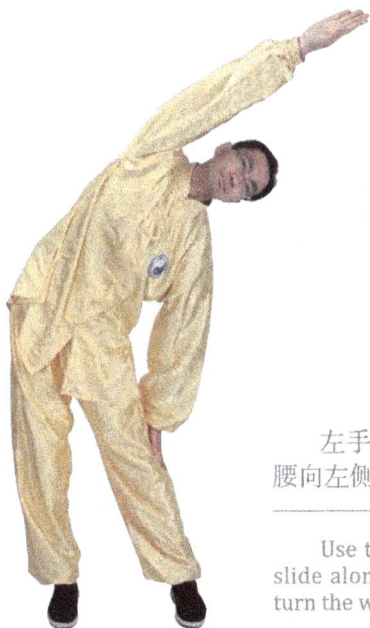

左手中指沿左侧中线大腿下滑，同时腰向左侧弯曲。

Use the middle finger of the left hand to slide along the left midline of the thigh and turn the waist to the left.

图7-2　Fig 7-2

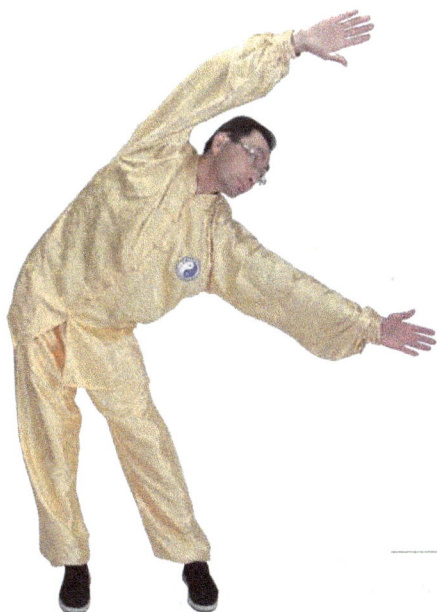

双手朝身体左侧伸展。

Extend the hands to the left.

图7-3　Fig 7-3

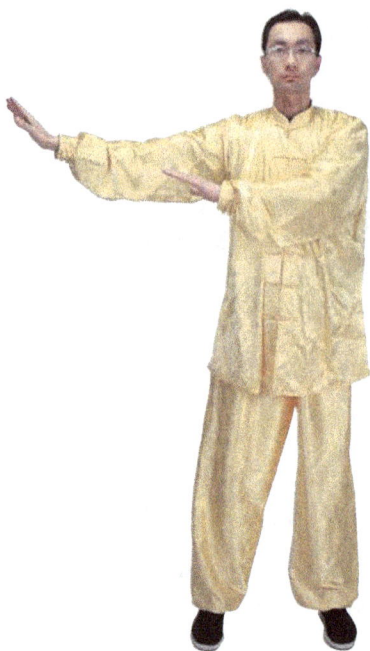

腰部逐渐伸直，双手上举，手心向前。两臂自然伸直，朝右侧下落至体前小腹下，手指垂地，两手心向内。

Slowly straighten up the waist and lift the hands (palms forward).Extend the arms and drop to the belly from the right side, making the fingers touch the floor, palms inward.

图7-4 Fig 7-4

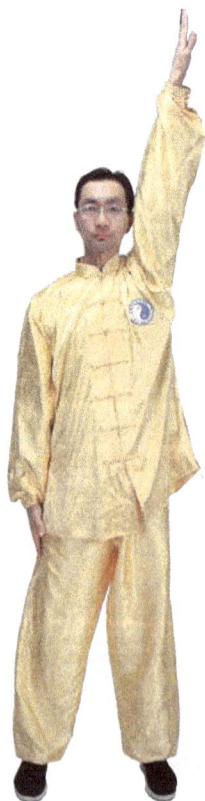

两臂由左侧缓缓上举，肘略曲，左臂贴耳，右臂下落，左掌心向外，指尖朝上。

Lift the arms from the left side of the body slowly. Slightly flex the elbows, make the left arm close to the ear and drop the right arm, making the palms outward and fingers pointing upward.

图7-5 Fig 7-5

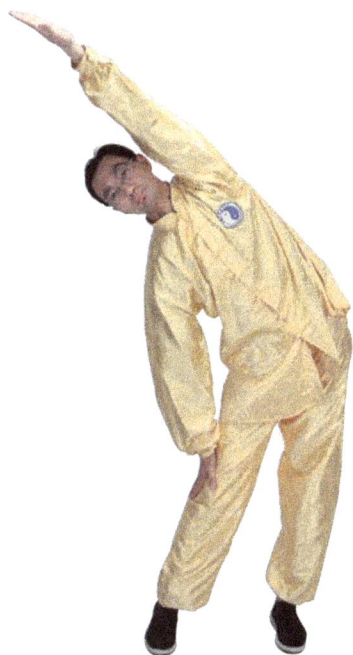

右手下落至右腿外侧
中线，中指沿右腿中线下
滑，同时，腰向右弯曲。

Drop the right hand to the
midline of the lateral aspect of
the right leg. Use the middle
finger of the right hand to
slide along the right midline of
the thigh and turn the waist to
the right.

图7-6　Fig 7-6

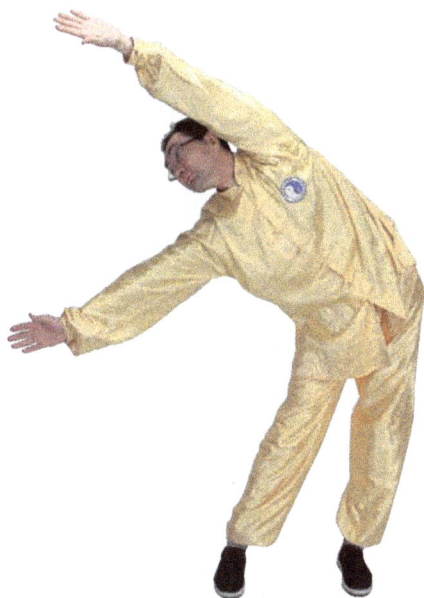

双手朝身体右侧伸展。

Extend the hands to the
right.

图7-7　Fig 7-7

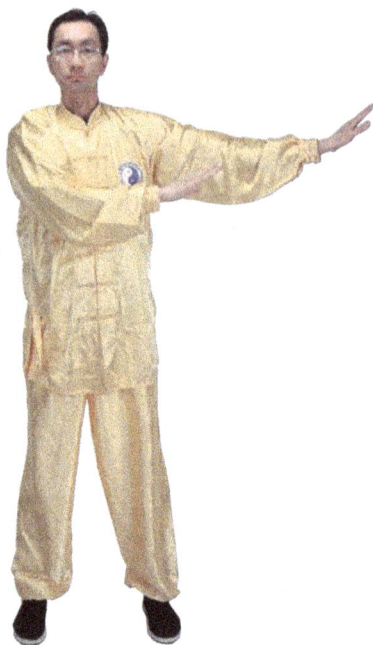

图7-8　Fig 7-8

　　腰部逐渐伸直，双手上举，手心向前。两臂自然伸直，朝左侧下落至体前，手指垂地，两手心向内。

　　Slowly straighten up the waist and lift the hands (palms forward).Extend the arms and drop to the front of the body from the left side, making the fingers touch the floor, palms inward.

本势动作左右各习练3次。

Repeat 3 times on each side.

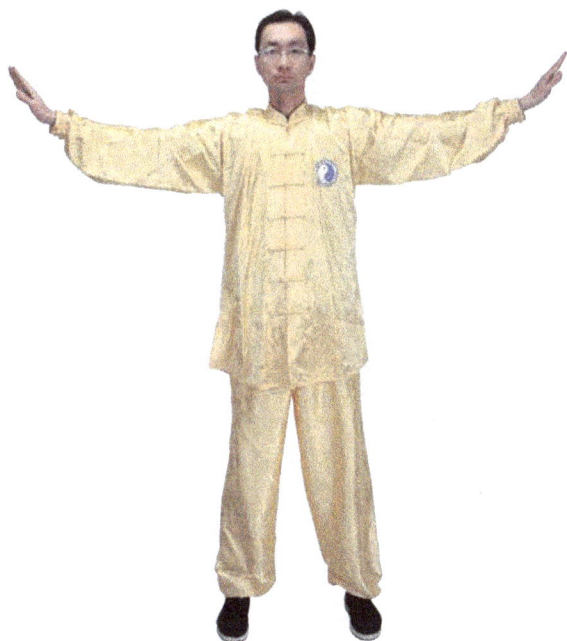

图7-9   Fig 7-9

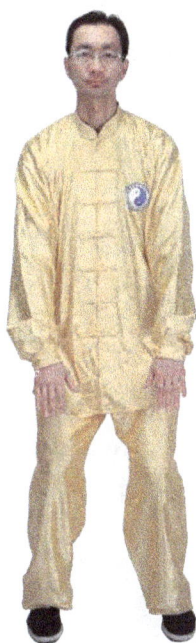

图7-10   Fig 7-10

结束时，两臂上举至头顶上方，双手分别由身体两侧至大腿前，掌心向下（图7-9、图7-10）。

Conclusion: Lift the arms above the top of the head and place the hands from both sides of the body to the front of the thighs, palms downward. (Fig 7-9, Fig 7-10)

2. 调息
2. Regulating the breathing

呼吸自然,吸气时动作向上,呼气时动作向下。

Natural breathing. Inhale while lifting movements and exhale with dropping movements.

3. 调心
3. Regulating the mind

意念专注于两掌。

Focus the mental concentration on the palms

[操作提示]

双手臂在练习过程中注意一手沉肩垂指,一手举臂伸指,两足可平行分开略宽于肩。

[Tips]

Use one hand to relax the shoulder and drop the fingers, use the other hand to lift the arm and extend the fingers. Place the feet slightly wider than the shoulder-width.

第八势　按摩丹田
Movement # 8 Massage Dantian

1. 调身
1. Regulating the body

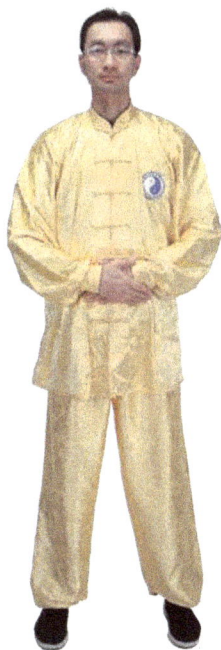

接上势，双目平视，双腿慢慢站直，双手从大腿前上提至腹部，双手掌相叠（男左手在内，女右手在内），轻轻按于脐中，然后按上、左、下、右，即顺时针方向按摩9圈。

Further to the last movement, look straight ahead, slowly stand up, and lift the hands from the front of the thighs to the level of abdomen. Overlap the palms (left hand inward for men and right hand inward for women) and gently press the umbilicus and massage 9 times clockwise.

图8-1　Fig 8-1

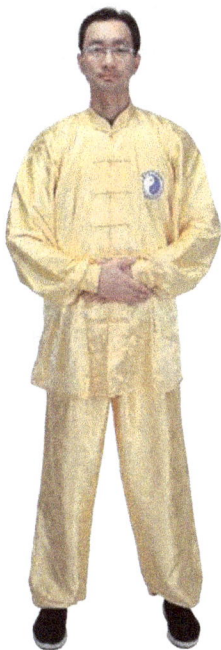

双手掌相叠至小腹前，然后按上、右、下、左，即逆时针方向按摩9圈。

Place the overlapped palms on the front of the abdomen and massage 9 times counterclockwise.

图8-2　Fig 8-2

2. 调息

2. Regulating the breathing

自然呼吸。

Natural breathing.

3. 调心

3. Regulating the mind

意念轻轻地守于丹田或掌心劳宫。

Focus the mental concentration on Dantian or Laogong[1] (PC 8).

[操作提示]

习练时，身体自然站立，凝神定志，动作轻柔而舒缓。

按摩动作连贯如画圆，以脐为中心，上不过膻中，下至小腹。

[Tips]

During exercise, keep the body upright, have a tranquil concentrated mind and conduct soft easy movements.

Massage is centered on the umbilicus. Do not go past Danzhong (Ren 17) and the lower abdomen.

---

1. Location: At the centre of the palm, between the 2nd and 3rd metacarpal bones, but close to the latter, and in the part touching the tip of the middle finger when a fist is made.

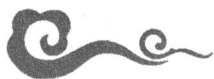

松 柔 功 • *Song Rou Gong* (Soft and Relaxed Exercise)

Application

应用

功　　理

Mechanism

　　导引，"导"古代作疏通、宣导解。"引"有伸展、引使之意。《灵枢·官能》上说："理血气而调诸逆顺，察阴阳而兼诸方，缓节柔筋而心和调者，可使导引行气。"因而导引有调节气血的保健作用。本功法就是通过形、意、气的导引，重点锻炼脊柱、四肢和心、肝、脾、肺、肾功能，以达到疏通经络、协调脏腑、调和气血，有病防病、无病强身的目的。以下简要介绍一下"松柔功"的机制。

As for *Dao Yin*, the first word *Dao* means to dredge and guide and the second word *Yin* means to stretch and pull. The *Ling Shu Guan Neng Pian* (chapter 73 of the Spiritual Pivot) states, '... can be treated with acupuncture harmonize qi and blood and observe the abundance or insufficiency of yin and yang; those with flexible joint movements and a peaceful mind can be treated with *Dao Yin* (guiding and stretching) to circulate qi'. Through *Dao Yin* of the body, mind and qi, *Song Rou Gong* in this text aims to exercise the spine, four limbs and functions of the heart, liver, spleen and kidney to unblock meridians, harmonize qi and blood of the zang-fu organs and promote health. The mechanism of *Song Rou Gong* is explained as follows:

形体导引——以发动气机为主，疏通经络，提高平衡人体气血阴阳的能力。

Dao Yin movements of the body

Purpose: to active qi activity, unblock meridians, harmonize qi and blood and balance yin and yang.

  "松柔功"的形体导引动作是根据人体上、下、左、右、前、后六个不同运动方向进行的。其动作的变化,始终按照人体"气机"的特定运行规律——升降、开合、出入等状态展开。功法的每个动作都在形体的相应部位产生一松一紧、升降开合、前后出入以及太极弧形、太极抱球等变化。这样的动作变化能有效地加快全身血液循环,促进人体新陈代谢,使人体全身的气机通和调顺。以本功法第一、第二节为例,这两节的动作要求以两手带动机体的上下升降起伏,以及胸前膻中上、下、左、右的开合,同时结合良性的意念活动,便能有效调节十二经脉指趾末端的穴位和全身气机,推动全身经络气血的流畅,从而最大限度地调动和保持机体内外的阴阳动态平衡,即达到中医所说的"阴平阳秘,精神乃治"的境界。故长期坚持习练"松柔功",可以调节人体气机,使之升降有序,出入有度,从而保证内气的各种生理功能得以充分发挥,使人体的生命活动正常进行,既保证了人体对营养物质的充分吸收,又能使体内代谢产物尽快排除,从而增进体力,提高健康水平。

Dao Yin movements of the body are performed in six directions (upward, downward, left, right, back and front). All movements are based on specific circulation of qi — ascending, descending, opening, closing, entering and exiting. Each movement produces relaxing, tightening, ascending, descending, opening, closing, entering, exiting, Taiji arch and balloon-holding in corresponding body parts. These movements can effectively accelerate blood circulation, facilitate metabolism and unblock and harmonize qi activity within the body. For example, movement # 1 and 2 use both hands to guide ascending and descending of the body and opening and closing of the chest [Danzhong (Ren 17)]. This, coupled with positive mental intent, can regulate *jing*-well points (located on the tips of the fingers or toes) of the twelve regular meridians, activity qi activity of the whole body and thus maximally balance yin and yang. Consequently, persistent practice of *Song Rou Gong* can regulate qi activity, guarantee normal functioning of internal qi (to secure full absorption of nutrients and remove metabolic wastes), increase physical strength and promote health.

意念导引——以良性意念为主，消除紧张状态，提高人体身心的协调能力。

Dao Yin of the intent

Purpose: to release stress with positive thinking and increase the coordination of body and mind.

"松柔功"的意念活动的特点是，轻松愉快，悠然自得且无限美好，例如意想大自然美景或其他美好的事物，倾听远处树林的鸟鸣声、流水声等。开始练功时首先把许多负面的情绪排除在头脑之外，替而代之以上述的良性意念，以此来消除各种杂念的干扰并缓解各种生理与病理性的紧张状态，降低对外界不良刺激的反应程度。同时练功者通过意守体内某一部位或某一体窍，例如意想或意守丹田、命门、劳宫、涌泉等穴位，可主动放弃日常之思虑活动，排除思想杂念，集中注意力来关注身体内部的气血运行，诱导大脑入静，使身体放松，处于气血融融、活泼自在的内外协调统一状态。这一状态使大脑皮层活动受到抑制，全身骨骼肌肌张力下降，大脑皮质下中枢自律调节，通过自主神经使分布广泛的脏腑功能协调统一。处于这种状态下，人体神经——内分泌按自然节律活动，平滑肌（包括心肌）按自然规律收缩与舒张，推动体液自然循环，物质能量自然代谢。这样一来，人体的生理、生化过程便处于最优状态，大脑皮层对整体的应激性反应得到缓解，对不良情绪的控制能力增强，为机体休

整、恢复提供有利条件，最终达到增进健康的目的。

Mental intent of *Song Rou Gong* is characterized by carefree, unhurried and infinite beauty. For example, you can imagine beautiful scenes or other nice things or listening to bird twittering and water flowing in the woods. When you start to practice *Song Rou Gong*, replace all negative ideas with above positive imaginations. This can help to remove distracting thoughts, alleviate physiological or pathological stress and minimize reaction to pessimal external stimulation. At the same time, you can also focus you mental intent on certain body parts, such as Dantian, Mingmen[1], Laogong (PC 8) and Yongquan (KI 1). This can help you to remove distracting thoughts and concentrate on internal circulation of qi and blood, thus obtaining a relaxed harmonious state. This state can inhibit the cerebral cortex activity, decrease skeletal muscle tension, regulate the autonomic nerve and harmonize functions of zang-fu organs. In this state, you can obtain natural rhythm of nerve-endocrine, natural contraction and relaxation of smooth muscles, natural circulation of body fluids and natural metabolism of matter energy. This is an optimal state of physiological and biochemical process. This state can alleviate stress reaction of the cerebral cortex, control unhealthy emotions, benefit body recuperation or recovery and promote health.

呼吸导引——以平和的自然呼吸为主，结形体导引、意念导引有效提升各脏腑的功能。

Dao Yin of breathing

Purpose: to combine natural breathing with Dao Yin of the body and mind to improve functions of the zang-Fu organs.

---

1. Mingmen literally means the gate of life, located between the kidneys, at the level of the second lumbar vertebrae.

　　松柔功的呼吸锻炼，初学时应强调平和缓慢的自然呼吸，以加强松静的效应。同时，由于主动进行身体放松与精神入静，使身心均处于松弛安静的状态，因此呼吸更易平稳通畅。通过一个阶段练习后，练功者的呼吸频率自然逐渐减慢，呼吸中枢的功能逐步得到改变和调整。随着练功的深入，应在意念的支配下，主动吸收自然界的新鲜氧气，清除体内的浊气、废气，并有意识地调整呼吸，使之逐步变得缓慢、深长、细匀。而缓慢深长的腹式呼吸对自主神经系统有明显的调整作用，因此能调整和强化各脏腑的活动功能。本功法的呼吸导引方法，始终与形体、意念导引相结合，体现以形导气，以意行气的呼吸形式。例如第三节的抱球托天、第四节的转体推掌和第五节的拗身回望，其呼吸导引方法既有平吸平呼，又有腹式呼吸。在呼吸过程中体内腰肌、腹肌、横膈肌进行升降、左右旋转的活动，这便直接对腹腔各内脏起到良好的按摩作用，从而改善和促进胃肠的血液循环与胃肠的蠕动，加强消化系统的功能。故练功后，食欲有所增加，面色渐趋红润。体力亦随之增进，达到协调脏腑，充实和培育人体内气，增进健康的目的。

　　It's advisable for beginners to use natural slow and gentle breathing to strengthen the relaxation and tranquil. At the same time, a relaxed and tranquil state of both body and mind makes breathing easier. Over time, along with the slowing down of respiration rate and improvement of the respiratory center, one needs to use intent to actively breathe in fresh oxygen and breathe out turbid qi, enabling the breathing to be slow, deep and even. Slow deep abdominal breathing can significantly regulate autonomic nervous system and thus boost the functions of zang-fu organs. Breathing in Song Rou Gong is always integrated with body movements and mental intent (i.e., use body movements to guide qi and use intent to circulate qi). For example, movement # 3 (hold a balloon to lift the sky), 4 (turn the body to push the palms) and 5 (turn the body to look back) contain both natural breathing and abdominal breathing. During respiration, ascending, descending and left-right rotation of lumbar, abdominal and diaphragmatic muscles directly massage abdominal organs, improve gastrointestinal blood circulation, increase gastrointestinal motility and benefit the digestive system. As a result, practice of *Song Rou Gong* can increase appetite, beautify the facial complexion, harmonize zang-fu organs, cultivate and supplement internal qi and promote health.

总之, 本功法是以形体导引为基础, 以良性意念调节为主导, 以与形体、意念导引相结合的自然轻柔的呼吸为推动力的一套整体养生功法, 在心理上可以调节改善人的紧张不安情绪与不良思维, 使人心情舒畅、朝气蓬勃、充满活力; 在生理上可进行整体性的自我调节, 有效地促进血液循环, 增强脏腑功能, 提高人体的适应能力和抵抗疾病的能力, 从而达到健身强体、防治疾病的目的。

In summary, *Song Rou Gong* is based on *Dao Yin* movements of the body, guided by positive mental intent and combined with natural breathing. Mentally, it can relieve stress, uneasiness and negative thinking, and obtain a happy mood and vitality. Physically, it can circulate blood, strengthen functions of zang-fu organs, increase adaptablity and disease-defending capability of the body and achieve health.

作 用

Functions

预备势: 通过松静站立, 以达到宁静心神, 调整呼吸, 内安脏腑, 外正身形。从精神与形体两方面做好练功前准备。

Through standing in tranquil and relaxation, the **preparation posture** helps to calm the mind, regulate breathing, harmonize the zang-fu organs and keep the body upright. This posture can help one to be well prepared physically and mentally.

展体舒气：通过双手的上升下降，身体的伸展和放松，可以发动真气，疏通经络，调和气血。人体之气通过上升下降在全身四肢运行。对于中老年人颈椎、腰椎关节病症及消化系统疾病有一定的防治作用。

Through ascending, descending, stretching and relaxing, **movement # 1** (stretch the body to soothe qi) activates genuine qi, unblock meridians, harmonize qi and blood and circulate qi flow through the four limbs and entire body. This movement can prevent and treat cervical or lumbar spondylosis and digestive disorders in the middle-aged and elderly people.

开阔胸怀：通过升降开合的运动，以升清降浊、调理气机，即把清阳之气引导于内，把浊阴之气导出体外，因此能加强肺部的气体交换，增强心肺的血液循环，增强胸肌、膈肌、腹肌运动。对心、肺疾病有一定的防治作用。

Through ascending, descending, opening and closing, **movement # 2** (open up the chest) ascends the clean (takes in the clean yang qi), descends the turbid (removes turbid yin qi) and regulates qi activity. This movement can enhance the gas exchange in the lungs, benefit cardiopulmonary blood circulation, exercise pectoral, diaphragmatic and abdominal muscles and prevent or treat cardiac or pulmonary conditions.

抱球托天：通过转腰及肢体上升下降的导引动作，重点锻

炼腰腹肌、膈肌、脘腹部肌肉,并对肝、脾、胃肠等内脏作轻柔按摩,具有健脾和胃、助消化作用,对胃肠疾病及自身脏腑功能低下的疾病有一定的康复保健作用。

Through turning the waist and ascending and descending movements of the limbs, **movement # 3** (hold a balloon to lift the sky) mainly exercises the abdominal, diaphragmatic and gastric muscles, and softly massage the liver, spleen, stomach and intestines. As a result, this movement can strengthen the spleen, harmonize the stomach, promote digestion and help to recovery from gastrointestinal disorders or hypo-functions of the zang-fu organs.

转体探掌:本式动作以内劲推掌为主,根基在脚,发力在腰,动作表现多在手掌。不仅能增强内劲,调和情志,扩大肺活量,增加体力,还能使人体的带脉得到疏通与调节,全身气机得以顺利升降。对中老年体虚、失眠和腿脚无力具有一定的保健康复作用。

Although manifesting in the palms, the root of **movement # 4** (turn the body to push the palms) is the feet, the internal strength (force) is from the waist. This movement can increase internal strength, regulate emotions, increase the lung capacity, unblock Dai[1] meridian and circulate qi activity of the entire body. Practice of this movement can benefit fragility, insomnia and leg weakness in the elderly.

拗身回望:通过左右转身回望,伸展两臂的动作,可增强腰肌、韧带的活动力度,使脊柱的功能得到改善或强化。对中老年腰背酸痛、关节错位和外感风寒具有一定的保健康复作用。

---

1. One of the eight extraordinary meridians that goes round the waist like a belt binding the yin and yang meridians.

Through stretching the arms and turning to left or right to look back, **movement # 5** can increase the activity of lumbar muscles and ligament and thus benefit the spine. Practice of this movement can benefit low back soreness and pain, subluxated joints and external contraction of wind-cold in the middle-aged and elderly people.

双手举鼎：通过以"内劲"来抓拳提升、上举下按，可加强全身脏腑或功能和血液循环。具有调整全身气机，通调水道，梳理上、中、下三焦之气的作用。对消化性溃疡有一定疗效。

Through lifting and pressing fists with internal strength, **movement # 6** (lift the tripod with both hands) can circulate blood, strengthen zang-fu functions, regulate qi activity of the upper, middle and lower *jiao*, and unblock water passage. Practice of this movement is beneficial for peptic ulcer.

左右侧弯：通过对腰背部及上肢肌肉的牵拉，可缓解腰背酸痛、肩关节疼痛。长期习练可壮筋骨，增强四肢力量。对胸椎、腰椎疾病有一定疗效。

Through pulling and stretching the lumbar, back and upper limb muscles, **movement # 7** (bend to the left and right) can alleviate soreness and pain in the low back and shoulder. Practice of this movement can strengthen the tendons and bones, increase strength of the four limbs and benefit thoracic and lumbar spondylosis.

按摩丹田：通过双掌按摩腹部，可调节肠胃功能，并帮助气息归根，气沉丹田，增补元气。对消化不良、便秘有一定疗效。

Through massaging the abdomen with both palms,

movement # 8 (massage Dantian) can regulate the stomach and intestines, return qi to its origin, help qi to sink to Dantian and thus supplement yuan-primordial qi. Practice of this movement can benefit dyspepsia and constipation.

Through tapping the body, the **concluding posture** can bring the person who practices qigong back to the normal state.

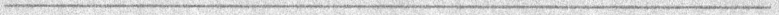

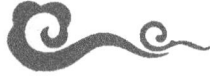

松 柔 功 ● *Song Rou Gong* (Soft and Relaxed Exercise)

The Meridian Charts

经络图

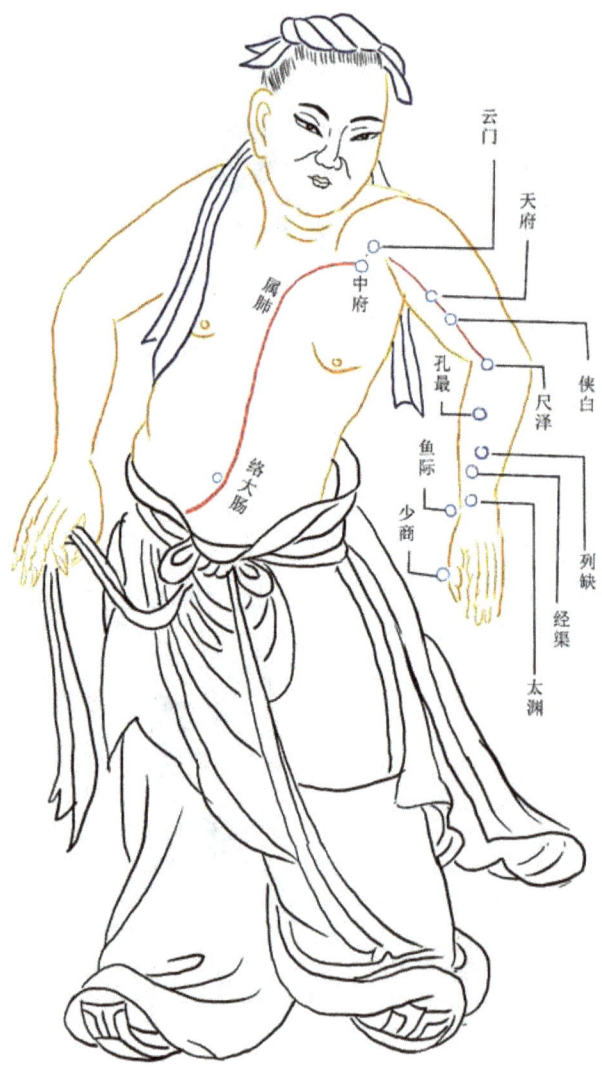

云门
天府
侠白
尺泽
孔最
列缺
经渠
太渊
鱼际
少商

属肺
中府
络大肠

手太阴肺经

Lung Meridian of Hand-Taiyin

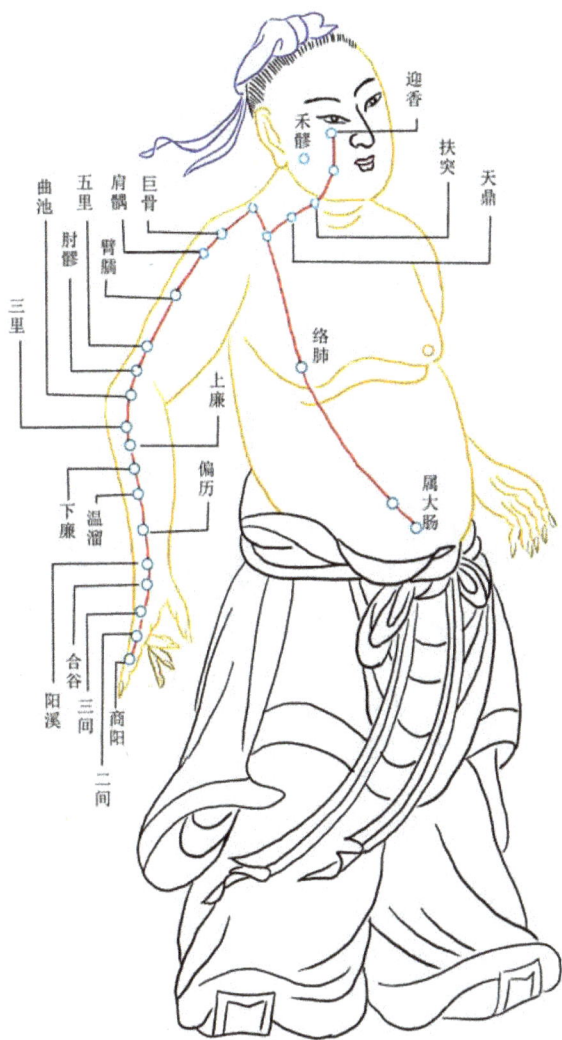

迎香
禾髎
扶突
天鼎
络肺
属大肠

曲池
五里
肩髃
巨骨
肘髎
臂臑
三里
上廉
偏历
下廉
温溜
合谷
三间
阳溪
商阳
二间

手阳明大肠经

Large Intestine Meridian of Hand-Yangming

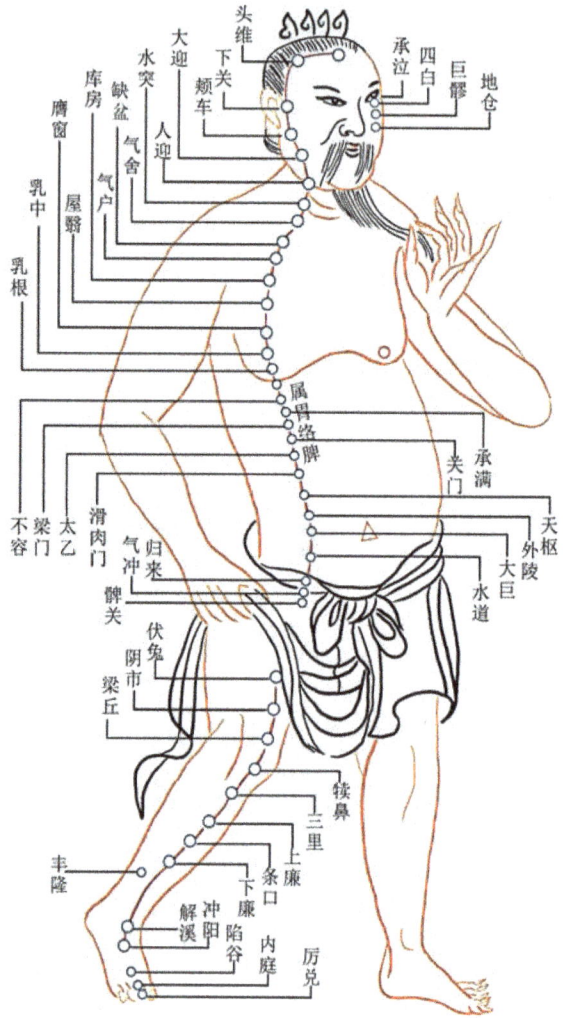

头维
下关
颊车
人迎
缺盆
气舍
气户
气舍
气户
屋翳
乳中
乳根
大迎
水突
库房
膺窗
承泣
四白
巨髎
地仓

属胃络脾
承满
关门
天枢
外陵
大巨
水道

不容
梁门
太乙
滑肉门
气冲
归来
髀关
伏兔
阴市
梁丘

犊鼻
三里
上廉
条口
下廉
陷谷
内庭
厉兑
冲阳
解溪
丰隆

足阳明胃经

Stomach Meridian of Foot-Yangming

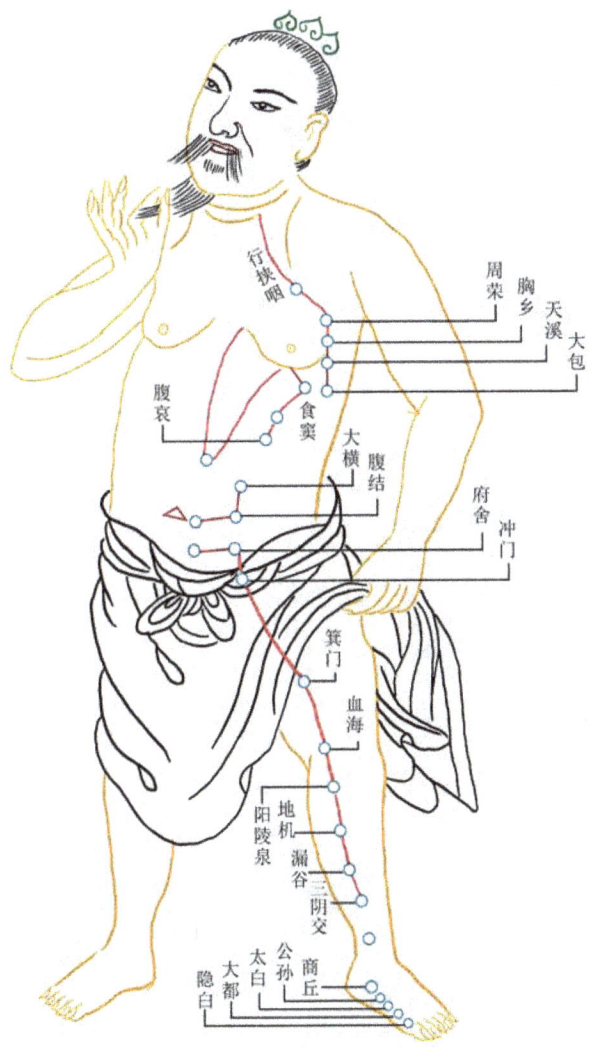

行挟咽
周荣
胸乡
天溪
大包
腹哀
食窦
大横
腹结
府舍
冲门
箕门
血海
地机
阳陵泉
漏谷
三阴交
公孙
商丘
太白
大都
隐白

足太阴脾经

Spleen Meridian of Foot-Taiyin

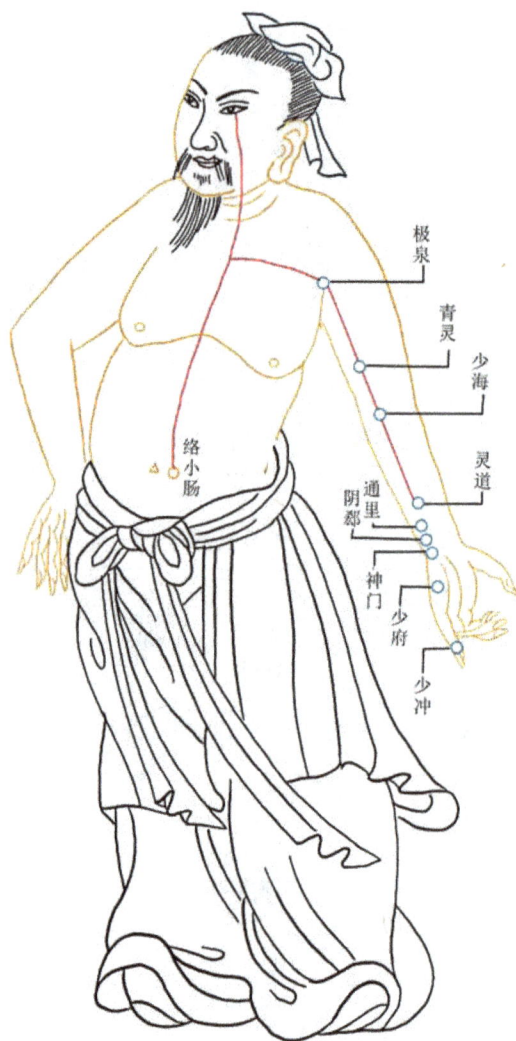

极泉

青灵

少海

灵道

通里
阴郄

神门

少府

少冲

络小肠

手少阴心经

Heart Meridian of Hand-Shaoyin

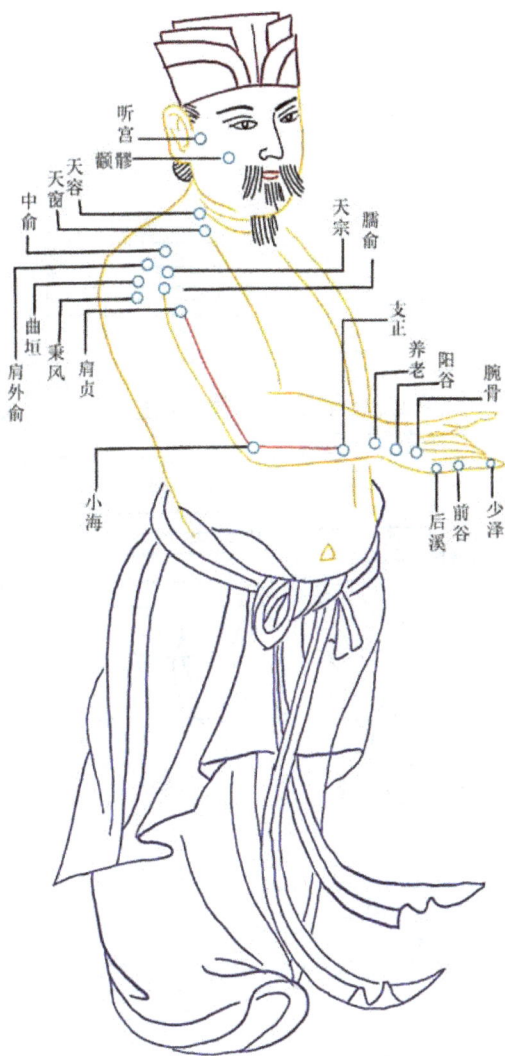

听宫
颧髎
天容
天窗
中俞
曲垣
秉风
肩贞
肩外俞
小海
天宗
臑俞
支正
养老
阳谷
腕骨
少泽
前谷
后溪

手太阳小肠经

Small Intestine Meridian of Hand-Taiyang

足太阳膀胱经

Bladder Meridian of Foot-Taiyang

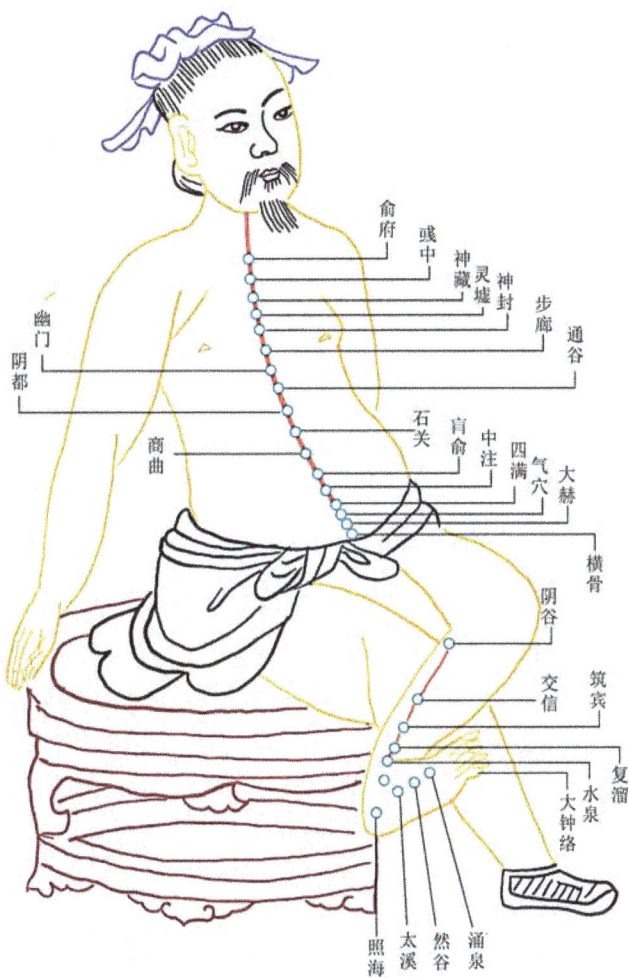

足少阴肾经

Kidney Meridian of Foot-Shaoyin

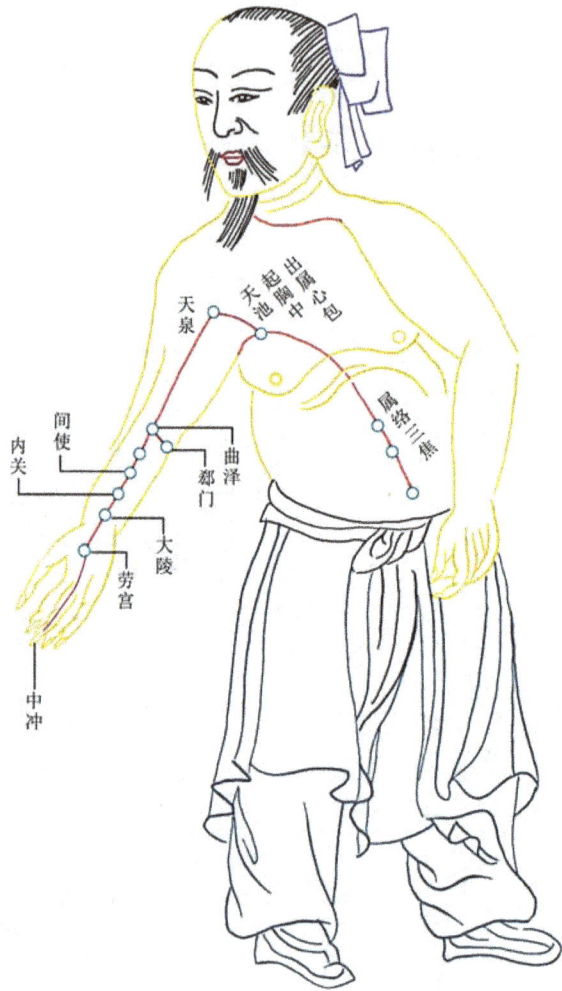

天泉
出属心包
起胸中
天池
属络三焦
间使
内关
曲泽
郄门
大陵
劳宫
中冲

手厥阴心包经

Pericardium Meridian of Hand-Jueyin

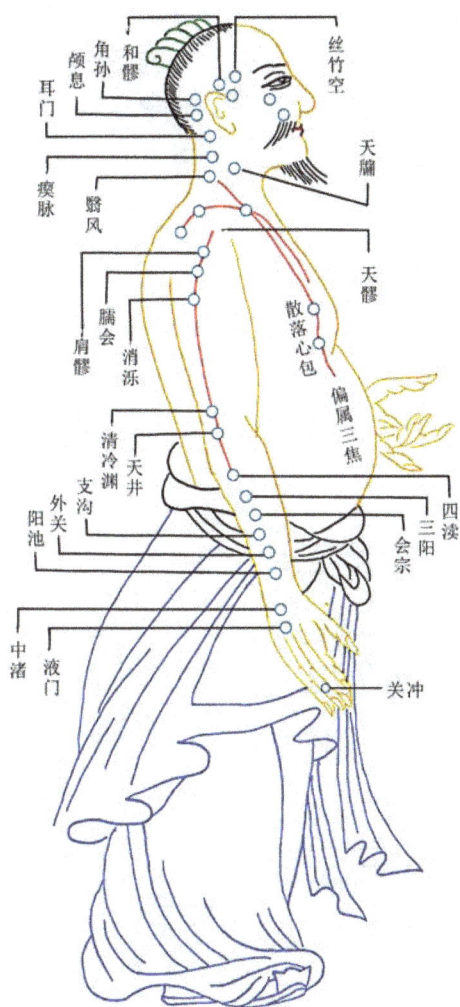

丝竹空
和髎
角孙
颅息
耳门
瘈脉
翳风
天牖
臑会
肩髎
消泺
天髎
散落心包
偏属三焦
清冷渊
天井
支沟
外关
阳池
四渎
三阳
会宗
中渚
液门
关冲

手少阳三焦经

Triple Energizer Meridian of Hand-Shaoyang

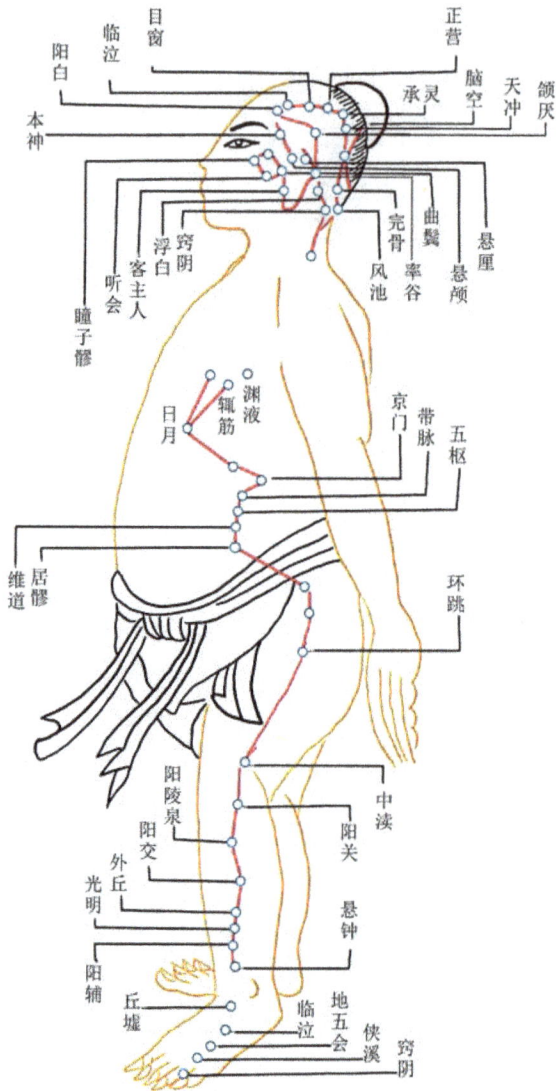

临泣　目窗　　　　　　正营
阳白　　　　　　　　　　　脑空　颔厌
　　　　　　　　承灵　天冲
本神
　　　　　　　　　　　　　悬厘
　　　窍阴　　　　　曲鬓　　悬颅
　　浮白　　　　完骨　率谷
客主人　　　　风池
听会
瞳子髎

　　　　　　渊液
　　　辄筋　　　京门　带脉
日月　　　　　　　　五枢

　　　　　　　　　　　环跳
　居髎
维道

　　　　　　　　中渎
阳陵泉
阳交　　　　阳关
外丘
光明　　　　　悬钟
阳辅
　丘墟　　临泣　地五会
　　　　　　　侠溪　窍阴

足少阳胆经

Gallbladder Meridian of Foot-Shaoyang

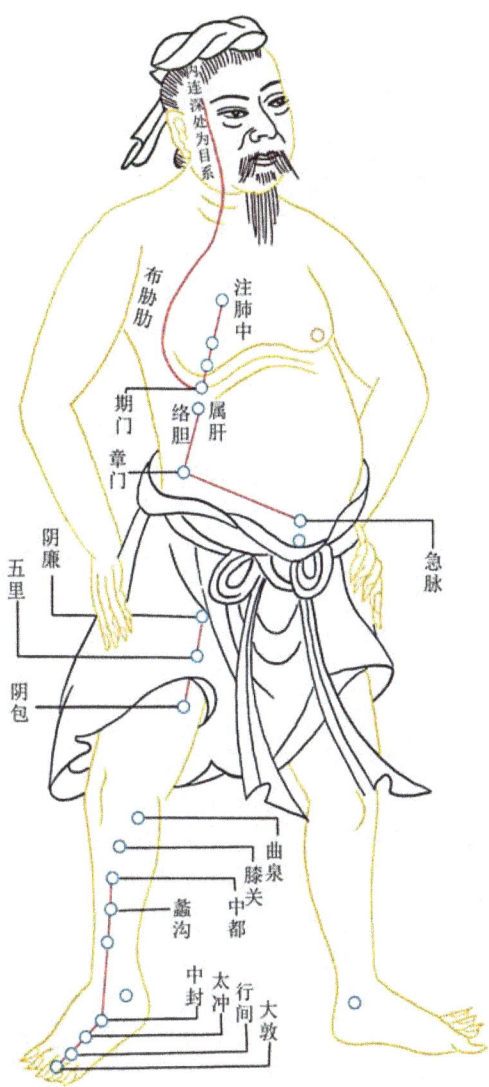

足厥阴肝经

Liver Meridian of Foot-Jueyin

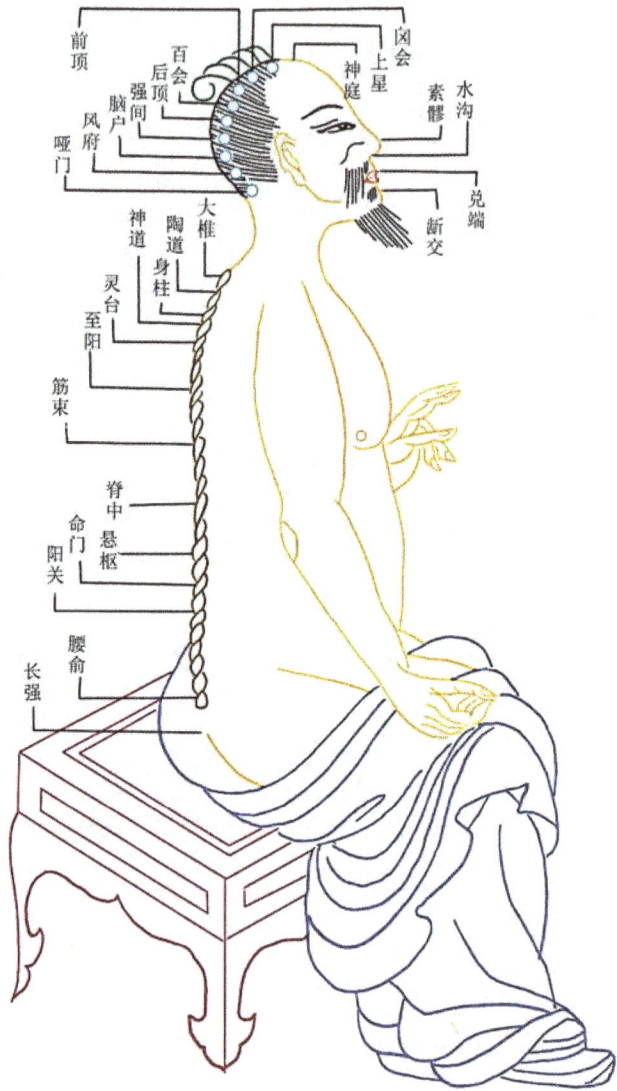

前顶
百会
后顶
强间
脑户
风府
哑门
囟会
上星
神庭
素髎
水沟
兑端
龈交
大椎
陶道
神道
身柱
灵台
至阳
筋束
脊中
悬枢
命门
阳关
腰俞
长强

督脉

Governor Vessel (Du)

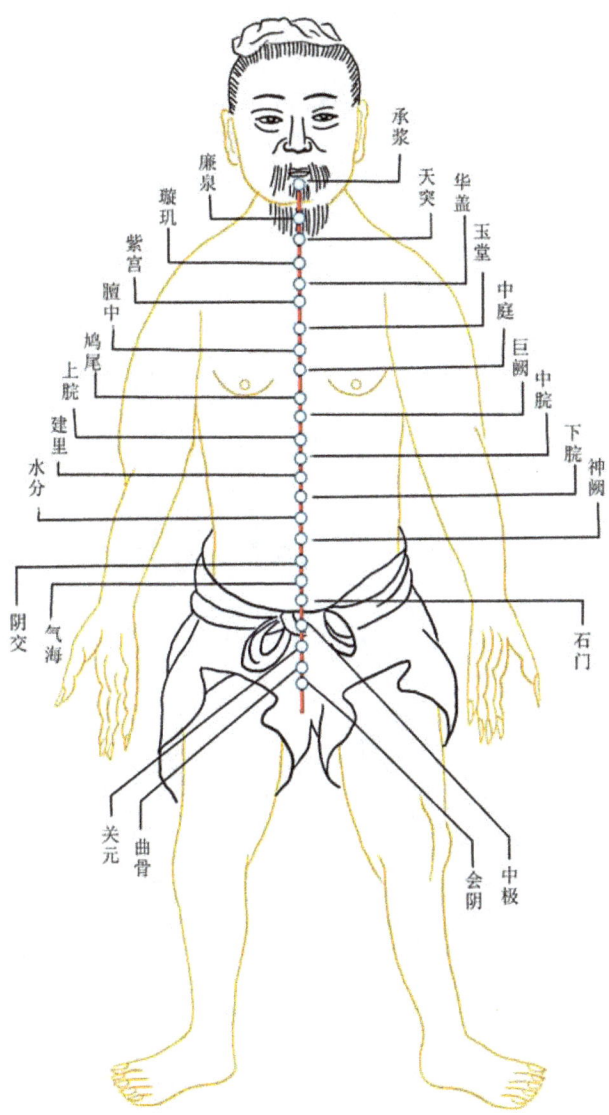

承浆
廉泉
璇玑
紫宫
膻中
鸠尾
上脘
建里
水分
阴交
气海
天突
华盖
玉堂
中庭
巨阙
中脘
下脘
神阙
石门
关元
曲骨
会阴
中极

任脉

Conception Vessel (Ren)

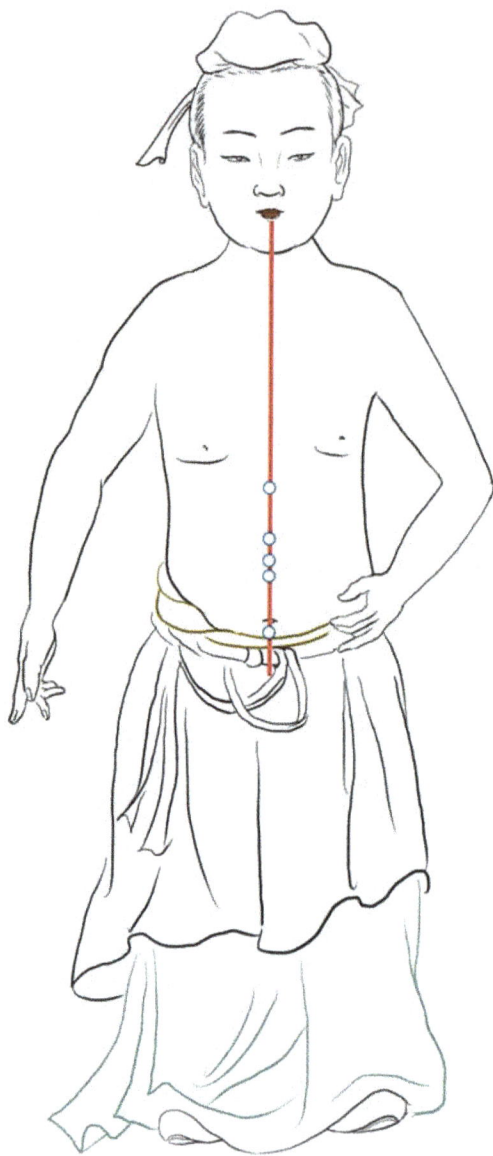

冲脉

Thoroughfare Vessel (Chong)

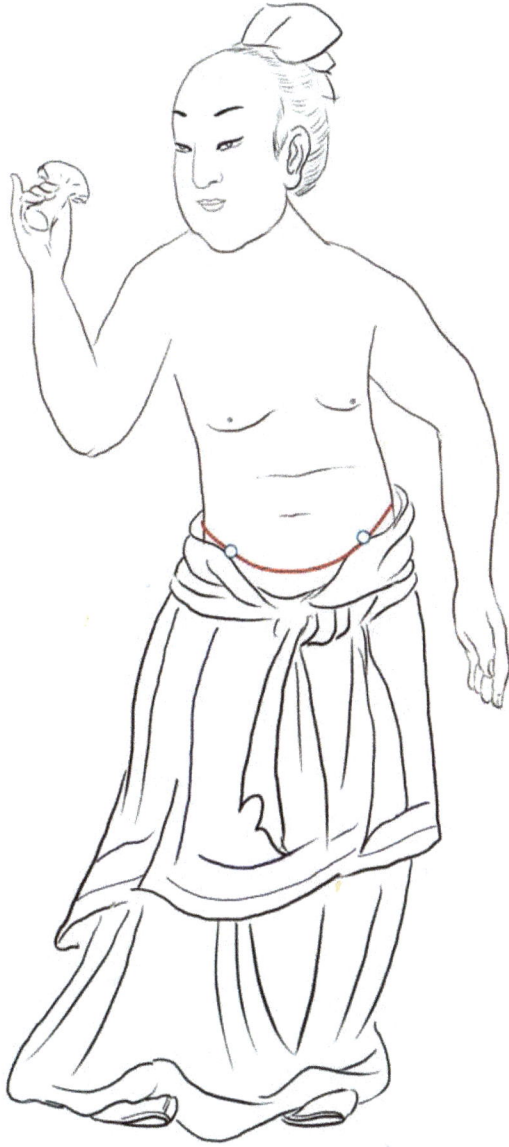

带脉

Belt Vessel (Dai)

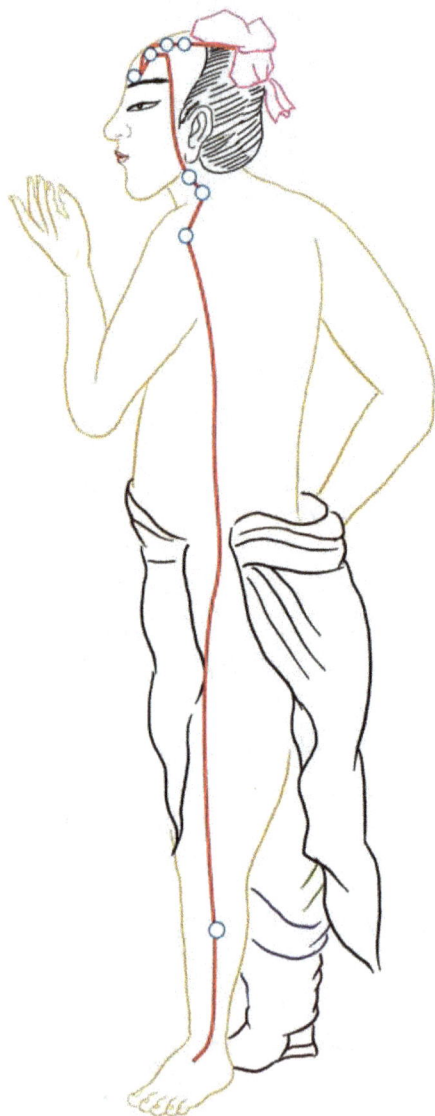

阳维脉

Yang Link Vessel (Yang Wei)

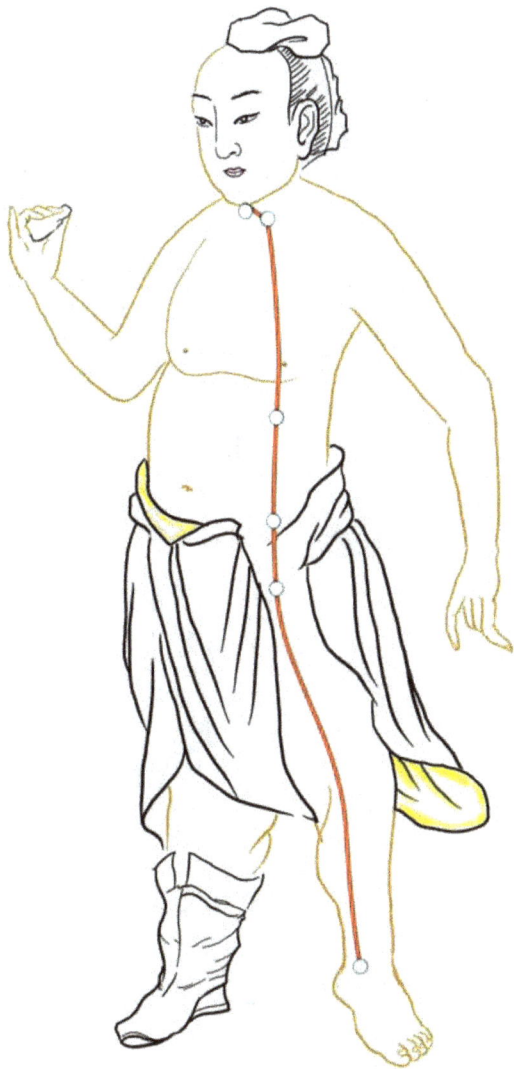

阴维脉

Yin Link Vessel (Yin Wei)

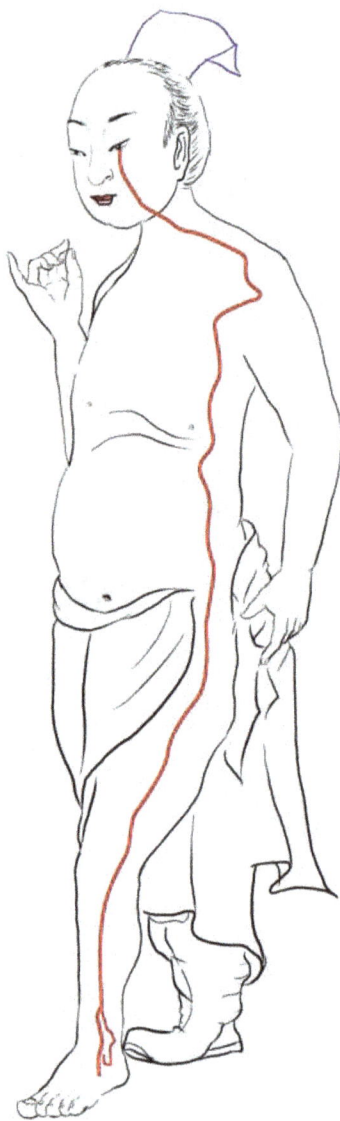

阳蹻脉

Yang Heel Vessel (Yang Qiao)

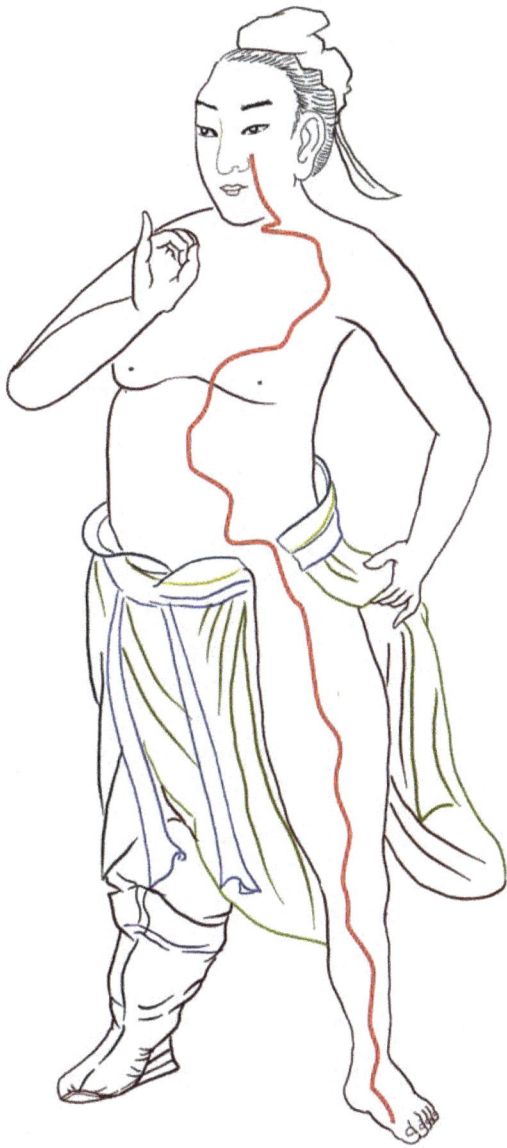

阴蹻脉

Yin Heel Vessel (Yin Qiao)

www.ingramcontent.com/pod-product-compliance
Lightning Source LLC
Chambersburg PA
CBHW081418270326
41931CB00015B/3324